More Praise for *100 Questions & Answers About Adult ADHD*

"Although adult ADHD is often a misunderstood and perplexing condition, readers may well find that they no longer have questions about adult ADHD after reading this book! Ava Albrecht, MD, has a masterful command of this subject yet she writes in a practical, straightforward, and 'user-friendly' manner, making this a highly recommended resource. For any adult who has been wrongly characterized as 'lazy,' 'disorganized,' 'lacking focus,' or 'spaced-out,' when attention-deficit issues were the real culprit, this volume will come as a welcome source of comfort and understanding. Dr. Albrecht, a voice of authority based on her prior well-respected books about depression and bipolar illness, offers in this volume her greatest contribution to date."

Sari Fine Shepphird, PhD
Clinical psychologist and author of
100 Questions & Answers About Anorexia Nervosa
Los Angeles, CA

100 Questions & Answers About Adult Attention-Deficit/ Hyperactivity Disorder (ADHD)

Ava T. Albrecht, MD

Clinical Assistant Professor of Child and Adolescent Psychiatry,
New York University School of Medicine
Service Chief, Adolescent Inpatient Unit,
Silver Hill Hospital
New Canaan, CT

JONES AND BARTLETT PUBLISHERS
Sudbury, Massachusetts
BOSTON   TORONTO   LONDON   SINGAPORE

World Headquarters

Jones and Bartlett Publishers
40 Tall Pine Drive
Sudbury, MA 01776
978-443-5000
info@jbpub.com
www.jbpub.com

Jones and Bartlett Publishers
Canada
6339 Ormindale Way
Mississauga, Ontario L5V 1J2
Canada

Jones and Bartlett Publishers
International
Barb House, Barb Mews
London W6 7PA
United Kingdom

Jones and Bartlett's books and products are available through most bookstores and online booksellers. To contact Jones and Bartlett Publishers directly, call 800-832-0034, fax 978-443-8000, or visit our website, www.jbpub.com.

Substantial discounts on bulk quantities of Jones and Bartlett's publications are available to corporations, professional associations, and other qualified organizations. For details and specific discount information, contact the special sales department at Jones and Bartlett via the above contact information or send an email to specialsales@jbpub.com.

Copyright © 2010 by Jones and Bartlett Publishers, LLC

All rights reserved. No part of the material protected by this copyright may be reproduced or utilized in any form, electronic or mechanical, including photocopying, recording, or by any information storage and retrieval system, without written permission from the copyright owner.

The authors, editor, and publisher have made every effort to provide accurate information. However, they are not responsible for errors, omissions, or for any outcomes related to the use of the contents of this book and take no responsibility for the use of the products and procedures described. Treatments and side effects described in this book may not be applicable to all people; likewise, some people may require a dose or experience a side effect that is not described herein. Drugs and medical devices are discussed that may have limited availability controlled by the Food and Drug Administration (FDA) for use only in a research study or clinical trial. Research, clinical practice, and government regulations often change the accepted standard in this field. When consideration is being given to use of any drug in the clinical setting, the healthcare provider or reader is responsible for determining FDA status of the drug, reading the package insert, and reviewing prescribing information for the most up-to-date recommendations on dose, precautions, and contraindications, and determining the appropriate usage for the product. This is especially important in the case of drugs that are new or seldom used.

Production Credits

Senior Acquisitions Editor: Alison Hankey
Editorial Assistant: Sara Cameron
Production Director: Amy Rose
Production Assistant: Laura Almozara
Senior Marketing Manager: Barb Bartoszek

Manufacturing and Inventory Control
  Supervisor: Amy Bacus
Composition: Appingo Publishing Services
Printing and Binding: Malloy, Inc.
Cover Printing: Malloy, Inc.

Cover Credits

Cover Design: Carolyn Downer
Cover Images: Top left: © Elena Ray/Shutterstock, Inc.; Top right: © Photodisc; Bottom: © Photos.com

Library of Congress Cataloging-in-Publication Data
Albrecht, Ava T.
  100 questions and answers about adult attention-deficit/hyperactivity
disorder (ADHD) / Ava T. Albrecht.
    p. cm.
  Includes bibliographical references and index.
  ISBN-13: 978-0-7637-5449-5
  ISBN-10: 0-7637-5449-8
  1. Attention-deficit disorder in adults—Miscellanea. I. Title. II.
Title: One hundred questions and answers about adult attention-deficit/hyperactivity
disorder (ADHD).
  RC394.A85A43 2010
  616.85'89—dc22
                        2008051160

6048

Printed in the United States of America
13 12 11 10 09   10 9 8 7 6 5 4 3 2 1

612.8589
A1b

DEDICATION

For Allison,
an inspiration for living.

GERMANTOWN COMMUNITY LIBRARY
GERMANTOWN. WI 53022

CONTENTS

As a Child and Adolescent Psychiatrist, I routinely deal with the diagnosis and treatment of Attention-Deficit/Hyperactivity Disorder (ADHD) in my work. Obtaining developmental and early childhood history is an important aspect to the evaluation of children and adolescents. In my work with adults, I carry this technique to those evaluations as well. In doing so, it has been clear that symptoms of ADHD that were present in childhood (whether diagnosed then or not) continue well into adulthood. The recognition of ADHD as a lifelong disorder came into being as I was moving out of adult psychiatric training into child and adolescent training. While ADHD has been recognized as a disorder that has been effectively treated for decades in children, it has continued to be surrounded in controversy, from beliefs of its overdiagnosis in children and theories of overmedicating our youth, to theories of adverse environmental conditions. It only follows that its recognition as a valid disorder in adults has been met with continued perpetration of misinformation in our society. But with misinformation also comes a greater willingness for individuals, such as well-known figures in popular culture, to share their personal histories, bringing forward greater understanding of the realities of living with ADHD. Increased media coverage both fosters increased education and facilitates the spread of myths. I have chosen to write this book because the recognition and understanding of ADHD as a lifelong condition is an important one. Symptoms can be easily mistaken for another condition, even by seasoned clinicians. When missed, lapses of appropriate treatment as well as the poor response of comorbid conditions can occur. Without a prior diagnosis, ADHD may not be of high consideration in adults presenting for treatment, but lack of a childhood diagnosis does not preclude diagnosis of ADHD in adults. In contrast to what some believe, ADHD is underdiagnosed in children and adolescents; thus, adults may present with symptoms for the first time in the context of a variety of difficulties that may not have developed if ADHD were recognized years earlier.

In my practice, I have seen many adults in whom ADHD was not picked up in childhood. It is missed for many reasons, one of which is the lack of early recognition of childhood psychiatric illness that occurred in earlier generations. Many of these adults were depressed or anxious, or abused substances in their youth. While these conditions may have occurred regardless of whether or not the ADHD was identified earlier, I cannot help but wonder if some of the difficulties later in life could have been avoided had the difficulties in childhood been recognized and treated. In many adults with whom I have worked, once the ADHD was identified and treated, comorbid conditions were often greatly alleviated or even resolved. The significance of untreated ADHD for many adults cannot be overestimated. Its treatment can bring an unexpected positive impact to people in their family and work lives. It can be a relief to know that the difficulties faced in childhood were not due to having been "dumb," "lazy," or an "airhead," or other unpleasant labels from society.

For me, the treatment of ADHD in adults is particularly gratifying because the impact of such treatment can be quite robust and can make significant improvements in the quality of life for many people. The benefits of feeling cohesive, organized, and productive cannot be overstated. Through this volume, it is my hope that a better understanding of this condition can be gained by both patients and their families, to help alleviate the stresses on relationships that can result in the presence of the sometimes chaotic, yet often exciting life of the person with ADHD.

Ava T. Albrecht, MD

Samantha Miller

Samantha Miller was diagnosed with ADHD at 45 years old, after her teenage daughter was diagnosed. Finding out that ADHD could possibly be at the core of her many problems was surprising. She wasn't easily convinced of having ADHD because she believed it to be a "fashionable" diagnosis for adults in 2005.

During subsequent months, while in graduate school studying to be a nurse practitioner, Samantha paid more attention to her thoughts and actions. She took note of her "frame of mind" and the impact of her symptoms on her life. Because she had worked the previous 23 years in medical-surgical nursing mostly in intensive care units, was obsessive and compulsive regarding schoolwork, and had a need for super-achievement that was reflected in studying around the clock since second grade, it was difficult for Samantha to believe she had ADHD.

Thinking about how she functioned throughout life, Samantha realized that ADHD symptoms were often at play. She notes being called many names in life: "the Taz," "road runner," "maniac," "bossy," "obnoxious," "pushy," and "mashuganah" (Hebrew for crazy). At the same time, she also realized that ADHD gave her an edge in many aspects of life. She could get an enormous amount done. Working as a waitress, she could serve twice as many tables. Her sometimes aggressive, pushy attitude, combined with a bubbly, convincing, and funny personality, always got her into places she wanted to be, including universities with scholarships and jobs for which she clearly was not prepared. But if she wanted something to happen, Samantha made it happen.

While she believes ADHD has provided her with many strengths through her impulsivity and hyperactivity, Samantha says she never feels normal. Even with all her Zen Buddhism teachings such as "there is no separateness," she still feels separate and different. With treatment, she has found a better ability to handle the stress of her world; however, she does not consider ADHD a hindrance. She finds that the power of a thousand thoughts per minute in stressful moments does need to be questioned, but those thoughts can be harnessed for their power. Now with psychiatric treatment, Samantha lives a joyful life. She can and does enjoy listening more while recognizing the chatter and repetition in her voice. She now recognizes and enjoys her silly sense of humor and accepts it as part of who she is.

Liza Miller

The summer following Liza's sophomore year in high school, at the age of 16, she attended a summer program at Pennsylvania State University. This was where her seemingly "psychotic" mental breakdowns officially began. What she remembers being so difficult for her was the fact that she had to live much more independently, both socially and, most of all, academically. Now, all she was to the teacher was a Social Security number and no longer a kind and innocent student who could fudge a few extra credit points. The stress of this experience led to the daily use of antacids and Prevacid, constant phone calls to her mother, and the onset of overwhelming feelings of sadness and uncertainty. Prior to that summer, her academic and social experiences were manageable, and Liza believed that, for the most part, she was very successful in both areas. Liza's grades were well above the norm, and she had been a part of a fun social circle. But college was different. College was real life.

In the fall of her junior year, Liza's mother brought her to an ADHD expert. The doctor asked many questions, and Liza filled out countless forms thinking, "Oh yes. . . definitely me." The inattentive symptoms had always been there, but Liza simply avoided them. Symptoms such as procrastinating, losing things constantly, having an embarrassing staring habit (that everyone seemed to notice), getting easily frustrated and irritated, driving too fast, being fidgety, finding it impossible to read a chapter or complete an assignment—the list went on and on. When the doctor asked, "Is it difficult to keep your ducks in a row?" Liza knew she really understood her dilemma.

A month or so after being prescribed Adderall, Liza felt the difference. Friends remarked that she no longer stared all the time. She could sit in a seat and take tests and focus better without realizing it. Her grades started to improve. But more importantly, her confidence started to improve. The anxiety lessened, and she felt that there was a better promise to her future college career.

Looking back on life—being placed in the slow reading group (second grade); having hysteria about long division (fourth grade); being incapable of finishing and understanding a book; and always feeling lost, stupid, and different from others, and confused about her own personal self—everything now makes sense to Liza. She recognizes how she had always compensated for her difficulties. Her mother worked with her—there were thousands of flash cards for every test. She received extra help before a test and got extra credit assignments to boost her grade after the tests, and teachers with whom she had close, friendly relationships had given her every opportunity to raise her grades.

Liza now attends a highly competitive university and studies in the library, giving herself plenty of time to prepare in an environment that helps her focus. Her social life is wonderful. She stopped smoking cigarettes and is very mindful of her alcohol consumption. She takes her medicine as prescribed. But, Liza admits. . . she still drives too fast.

PART ONE

The Basics

What is ADHD?

Is ADHD in adults a new diagnosis?

Is ADHD a psychiatric disorder or neurological disorder?

More ...

1. What is ADHD?

ADHD is the acronym for Attention-Deficit/Hyperactivity Disorder, which is a brain-based disorder that affects attention, motor activity, and impulse control. The major symptoms of the disorder are distractibility, forgetfulness, inability to concentrate, poor attention span, hyperactivity, and impulsiveness. While the term ADD is often used to describe Attention Deficit Disorder, strictly speaking ADHD is the correct medical term regardless of whether or not hyperactivity is present. Once considered a disorder of children and adolescents, ADHD is now recognized as a condition that typically persists into adulthood, with 65% to 85% of children who have ADHD continuing to meet full or partial criteria for ADHD as adults. Between 4% and 5% of the adult population in the United States is thought to be affected by ADHD, which translates to approximately 8 million adults with ADHD, most of whom are not treated. Many adults with ADHD are not aware they have the condition, due to the fact that its recognition as a disorder in adults is relatively recent. In the clinician's office, individuals often present with a variety of complaints and **functional** impairments, unaware that deficits in attention or impulse control have contributed to their problems. For example, individuals with ADHD have higher unemployment rates, a higher divorce rate, and higher risk for substance abuse. Since ADHD is a brain-based disorder, regions of the brain responsible for impulse control, planning, organization, and other **executive functions** appear to be involved. There is ample evidence for regional brain differences in persons with ADHD that supports the recognition of ADHD as a brain-based disorder that most often is a condition across the life span.

2. Is ADHD in adults a new diagnosis?

ADHD has long been considered a disorder of childhood and has an interesting history. It was recognized as early as 1902 when George Still, who noted people expressing symptoms of aggressiveness and defiance, and being overly emotional

---

Functional

Pertaining to the ability to perform day-to-day responsibilities, such as in one's work, home, and school lives.

Individuals with ADHD have higher unemployment rates, a higher divorce rate, and higher risk for substance abuse.

Executive functions

A set of cognitive abilities that control and regulate other abilities and behaviors.

and exhibiting cruelty toward others, described it as a "disorder of moral control." He specifically exempted cases related to a poor child-rearing environment, which highlights the recognition that it was a condition that arose independent of family environment. Following the encephalitis epidemic of 1917 to 1918, symptoms such as **hyperkinesis**, explosiveness, and attention deficit were noted in many children and were thus described in 1922 as a "post-encephalitic behavior disorder." In the late 1930s, symptoms of hyperkinesis, impulsivity, learning disability, and short attention span were described as the condition "minimal brain damage" and later as "minimal brain dysfunction" due to symptoms similar to those of brain-damaged patients, but in the absence of identifiable injury. Then, in 1960, Stella Chess described the "hyperactive child syndrome," which emphasized activity level as the defining feature, as well as specifically separating the condition from those arising secondary to brain damage, the prevailing notion in Europe at that time being that hyperkinesis was specifically due to brain damage. In 1968, the *DSM-II* first recognized this disorder as a "hyperkinetic reaction of childhood disorder."

In the *DSM-III*, the emphasis was moved from activity level to inattention as a significant component of the disorder. Symptoms were identified as due to Attention Deficit Disorder (with or without hyperactivity), and the qualifier "residual type" was introduced to describe remaining symptoms that continued to cause impairment. The *DSM-III-R* further defined the disorder, changing the name to Attention-Deficit/Hyperactivity Disorder and listing more specific symptoms. Criteria were further refined for the *DSM-IV*, which is described in Question 9. These criteria, however, did not serve to address symptoms that persisted beyond childhood.

While previously considered a disorder of childhood, with descriptors of the condition in the *DSM* specific to how symptoms manifest in children and adolescents, by the 1990s it was apparent that many children and adolescents continued to suffer from their ADHD symptoms well into adulthood.

Hyperkinesis
Hyperactivity; excessive motor movement.

The Basics

Mental illness

A medical condition defined by functional symptoms with as yet no specific pathophysiology that impairs social, academic, and occupational function.

Neurotransmitter

Chemical in the brain that is released by nerve cells to send a message to other cells via the cell receptors.

Neurological

Referring to all matters of the nervous system that include the brain, brainstem, spinal cord, and peripheral nerves.

Central nervous system

Nerve cells and their support cells in the brain and spinal cord.

Depression

A medical condition associated with changes in thoughts, moods, and behaviors.

Psychotic

Relating to the loss of contact with reality, which can be characterized by the presence of hallucinations or delusions.

With this recognition, there has been increasing amounts of research into the presentation of ADHD in adulthood. Increased research and increased media coverage on adult ADHD can make it appear to be a new diagnosis when, in fact, there is simply greater recognition within the medical profession that the condition has always existed.

3. Is ADHD a psychiatric disorder or neurological disorder?

As more and more evidence accumulates that **mental illness** is rooted in problematic brain functions, such as deficiencies in certain **neurotransmitters**, it becomes more difficult to clearly differentiate that which is mental from that which is **neurological**. In fact, while many mental illnesses are considered technically neurological, of and relating to the **central nervous system**, they are classified separately and treated by psychiatrists. Separation of psychiatric disorders from neurological disorders is arbitrary and not based upon scientific evidence. Similar to many psychiatric illnesses having neurological features, many neurological illnesses have psychiatric features, such as is seen in Parkinson's disease, which is commonly associated with dementia and **depression**. In dementia, a condition typically treated by neurologists, there can be various behavioral disturbances in patients as well as **psychotic** symptoms. The distinction between neurological and psychiatric disorders is based mainly upon historical and practical considerations. So, technically speaking, as the field of neurology treats brain diseases, at least the major mental illnesses that are rooted in abnormal brain functions could be called neurological disorders. The reality, however, is that illnesses such as schizophrenia, bipolar disorder, major depression, and so on continue to be regarded as mental illnesses, which are treated by psychiatrists and other mental health practitioners. These illnesses are thus listed and codified in the *DSM-IV-TR*, the current handbook on the treatment of mental disorders. Thus any condition in the handbook, including ADHD, would be considered a mental disorder that falls under the purview of psychiatric treatment. It is widely accepted, however, that ADHD is a **neurobiological** or neurological disorder, because numerous studies support its origin in the brain as well as its presence as a lifelong or **developmental disorder**. The inclusion of ADHD under the purview of psychiatric treatment likely stems from the behavioral components with which it often presents and its history of being considered a behavioral disorder. Behavioral disorders of any type often fall to the care of psychiatrists and other mental health care professionals. Many neurologists, however, particularly those who have specialized training in behavioral neurology, will treat ADHD, but they may be less inclined to do so in the presence of other psychiatric disorders. In addition, pediatricians will often treat uncomplicated ADHD in their patients. So ADHD can be considered a neurological disorder that falls primarily under the care of mental health clinicians, as do many behavioral disorders. As ADHD has a high **comorbidity** with many psychiatric disorders, its inclusion in the realm of mental health is certainly warranted.

4. What makes ADHD a neurobiological disorder?

While the condition is likely varied in its origins, much research has supported several neurobiological underpinnings of ADHD which include its **genetic** attribute. Research has found that in ADHD, various functions of the brain, such as **arousal**, sustained attention, executive functions, and **response inhibition** are impaired. ADHD is not a "made-up" or "fake" disorder, a function of "laziness," a result of poor parenting or lack of discipline, caused by a poor diet, nor is it commonly outgrown. **Neuroimaging** has revealed abnormalities in several regions of the brain including smaller brain volumes in all brain regions that persisted with age (and were unrelated to treatment with medication). In brain imaging studies that look at how brain areas respond to a specific stimulus, certain areas of the brain activate differently in adults with ADHD versus those without. Overactivity of a protein that transports dopamine has been found in ADHD adults, so that too much dopamine was carried from the synaptic cleft back to the **presynaptic** neuron.

The Basics

Neurobiological

Of or relating to the biological study of the nervous system.

Developmental disorder

One of several disorders that interrupt normal development in childhood.

Comorbid

The presence of two or more mental disorders, such as depression and anxiety.

Genetic

Of or relating to genes, the DNA sequence that codes for a specific protein or that regulates other genes. That which is genetic is heritable.

ADHD is not a "made-up" or "fake" disorder, a function of "laziness," a result of poor parenting or lack of discipline, caused by a poor diet, nor is it commonly outgrown.

Arousal

A state of responsiveness to sensory stimulation or excitability.

Response inhibition

In behavioral therapy, the weakening of a response to a given stimulus.

Neuroimaging

The use of techniques to create an image of the structure or function of the brain; CT scans and brain MRIs are examples.

Presynaptic

That part of a nerve cell that is proximal to the synapse.

Heritability

The proportion of observed variation of a particular trait that is attributable to genetic factors in contrast to environmental factors.

Gray matter

The part of the brain that contains the nerve cell bodies, including the cell nucleus and its metabolic machinery, as opposed to the axons, which are essentially the "transmission wires" of the nerve cell.

Additional support for the neurobiology of ADHD is provided by genetic studies that have found the average **heritability** to be 75%, a high rate in comparison to depression, for example. Genetic studies have implicated three dopamine genes that are connected to the symptoms of ADHD. Numerous studies demonstrate the connection between certain areas of the brain with the symptoms of ADHD, and research continues to better identify the specific deficits. It is likely that different patterns of abnormalities in the brain can lead to the symptom complex of ADHD and that different genes can be potentially involved in expression of the disorder.

5. How do chemicals work in the brain?

The brain is a complex organ that is comprised of **gray matter** and **white matter**. Gray matter consists of the cell bodies of **neurons** (**Figure 1**) and other support cells, and the white matter consists of long tracts of **axons** that run between the neurons. Different areas of the brain have somewhat specific functions. For example, the **motor cortex** controls voluntary movements of the body, and the sensory cortex processes information of the various sensory systems. Different areas of the brain communicate with other areas nearby as well as more distantly. Information travels via the axons of the neurons within the white matter areas of the brain.

The brain contains billions of neurons that interact with each other **electrochemically**. This means that when a nerve is stimulated, a series of chemical events occur that in turn create an electrical impulse. The resulting impulse propagates down the nerve length known as the axon and causes a release of chemicals called neurotransmitters into a space between the stimulated nerve and the nerve that it wishes to communicate with, known as the **synaptic cleft** (**Figure 2**). The neurotransmitters interact with **receptors** on the second nerve, either stimulating or inhibiting them. The interaction between the neurotransmitters and receptors can be likened to a key interacting with a lock where the neurotransmitter or "key" engages the receptor or "lock," causing it to "open." This

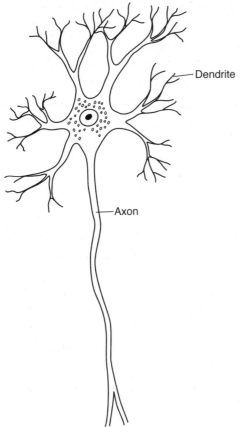

Dendrite

Axon

Figure 1   Neuron

The Basics

White matter

Tracts in the brain that consist of sheaths (called myelin) covering long nerve fibers.

Neuron

A nerve cell made up of a cell body with extensions called the dendrites and the axon. The dendrites carry messages from the synapse to the cell body, and the axon carries messages to the synapse to communicate with other nerve cells.

Axon

A single fiber of a nerve cell through which a message is sent via an electrical impulse to a receiving neuron.

Motor cortex

Portion of the cerebral cortex that is directly related to voluntary movement.

Electrochemically

The mechanism by which signals are transmitted neurologically. Brain chemicals, or neurotransmitters, alter the electrical conductivity of nerve tissue, causing a signal to be transmitted or sent.

opening is really a series of chemical changes within the second nerve that either causes that nerve to "fire" or "not fire." Thus, brain activity is the result of an orchestrated series of nerves firing or not firing in a binary fashion. In that sense, it is much like a computer in which very complicated processes begin their lives as a series of 1s or 0s (on or off, fire or do not fire).

After the nerve fires, thereby releasing neurotransmitters into the synaptic cleft, the neurotransmitters must be removed from the area in order to turn the signal off. There are two ways that these chemicals can be removed in order to turn the signal off. The first is by destroying the chemical through the use of another chemical known as an **enzyme** with that specific purpose in mind. The second is by pumping the chemical back

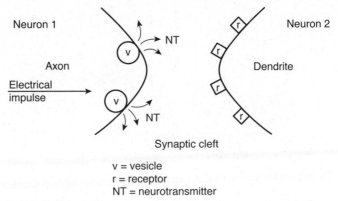

v = vesicle
r = receptor
NT = neurotransmitter

Figure 2 Synaptic Cleft

Synaptic cleft

The junction between two neurons where neurotransmitters are released, resulting in the transmission of a message between the two neurons.

All *psychoactive compounds, whether neurotransmitters, hormones, medications, or addictive drugs, involve one or more of these simple mechanisms.*

Receptor

A protein on a cell to which specific chemicals from within the body or from the environment bind in order to cause changes in the cell that result in an electrochemical message for a certain action to be taken by that cell.

into the nerve that released it by using another special chemical known as a **transporter** or transport pump. The process of pumping chemicals back into the nerve is known as **reuptake**. It is important to understand these basic principles of **neurophysiology** because *all* psychoactive compounds, whether neurotransmitters, hormones, medications, or addictive drugs, involve one or more of these simple mechanisms.

6. What chemicals in the brain are associated with ADHD?

There is considerable evidence that **norepinephrine** and **dopamine** are involved in attention, arousal, impulse control, and executive functioning, and the two are thought to collaborate in their functions. The theory that ADHD is a disorder of dopamine and norepinephrine is supported by the fact that medicine that is effective for ADHD symptoms acts primarily in dopaminergic and noradrenergic pathways and use of a medication that blocks dopamine receptors negates the actions of the medications. A hypothesis citing too much or too little of a given neurotransmitter in the brain as a cause of ADHD, however, is overly simplistic because the attention and arousal system in people is very complex. Dopamine and norepinephrine are very similar in structure, differing by one hydroxyl group (**Figure 3**), and are part of the group of chemicals called **catecholamines**. Catecholamines have been implicated in other psychiatric disorders, including depression

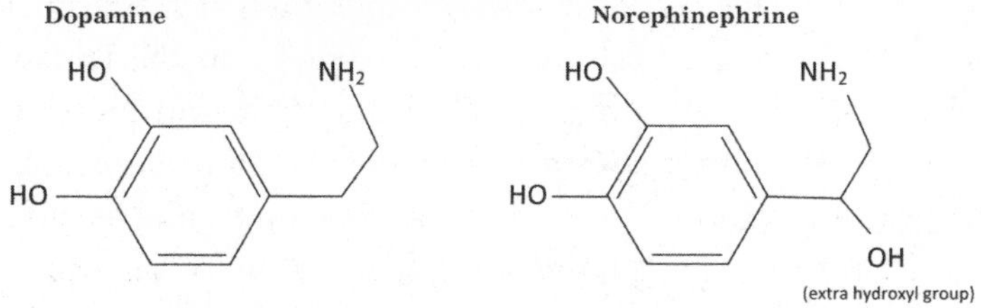

Figure 3   Dopamine and norepinephrine are very similar in structure, differing by one hydroxyl group.

and bipolar disorder. Dopamine is a precursor to the synthesis of norepinephrine in the brain, with both neurotransmitters present in varying amounts in different areas in the brain. Norepinephrine is generated from an area of the brain called the **locus ceruleus** with axons from this region projecting widely throughout the brain. This suggests that norepinephrine is a neuromodulator of sorts, meaning that it modulates the effects of other neurotransmitters in the brain. While it is not possible to completely separate the functions of the catecholamines in the brain, the role of norepinephrine is thought to include:

- The increase and maintenance of overall arousal
- Facilitation of emotional regulation related to response to danger or opportunity
- Facilitation of memory storage and retrieval

In the **peripheral nervous system**, norepinephrine prepares the body for the **fight-or-flight** response when confronted with danger. Affecting arousal, alertness, and activation within the brain enables an appropriate response to danger. Norepinephrine is also critical to executive functions as they relate to reasoning, learning, and problem solving.

Dopamine pathways in the brain arise from three regions of the **midbrain** and project axons through four main pathways to different parts of the brain that are responsible for intentional control of movement, the brain reward system, and motivational and emotional response areas. Dopamine

The Basics

Enzyme

A protein made in the body that serves to break down or create other molecules. Enzymes serve as catalysts to biochemical reactions in the body.

Transporter

A protein that travels through a cell membrane into a cell, carrying specific nutrients, ions, or chemicals with it.

Reuptake

The reabsorption of a substance by the cell that originally released the substance.

Neurophysiology

The part of science devoted specifically to the physiology of the nervous system.

Norepinephrine

A neurotransmitter that is involved in the regulation of mood, arousal, and memory.

Dopamine

A catecholamine that serves as a neurotransmitter in the brain.

Catecholamines

Amines that are derived from tyrosine and function as hormones, neurotransmitters, or both.

Locus ceruleus

An area within the brainstem with neurons that synthesize norepinephrine and from where axon projections spread widely throughout the central nervous system.

Peripheral nervous system

The part of the nervous system that constitutes nerves outside of the brain and the spinal cord, such as nerves that innervate the limbs.

Fight or flight

A reaction in the body that occurs in response to an immediate threat. Adrenaline is released, which allows for rapid energy to face the threat (fight) or run (flight).

in the frontal lobes controls the information flow from other parts of the brain. Problems with dopamine in the frontal lobes will adversely affect memory, attention, and problem solving. **Working memory** requires activation of dopamine receptors. Dopamine projections mediate prefrontal cortical processes that enable suppression of distractions or behavioral expressions to thoughts or ideas. In addition to its cognitive enhancing effects, dopamine is an integral part of the brain reward system.

7. What is executive functioning?

Executive functioning is the system within the brain that enables a person to control and firmly apply one's own mental skills. Many people with ADHD (but not all) have deficiencies in areas of executive functioning, which, in the human brain, appear to be mediated by the **prefrontal lobes** of the **cerebral cortex**. The executive functioning aspect of brain function was established upon observation of patients with frontal lobe brain injury. Patients with frontal lobe damage would exhibit disorganized functioning with everyday tasks, but paper and pencil tests would not reveal deficits in memory, learning, language, or reasoning. An "overseer" of basic cognitive processes was therefore thought to be part of the frontal lobe functions. Use of executive functioning allows us to identify a problem, make a plan, execute the plan, and then evaluate the outcome. Its area of the brain is our problem-solving center. Different aspects of executive function include: the ability to sustain or flexibly redirect attention, the inhibition of inappropriate behavioral or emotional responses, the planning of strategies for future behavior, the initiation and execution of these strategies, and the ability to easily switch among problem-solving strategies.

Additional roles of the "executive system" within the frontal lobes of the brain include involvement in processes such as planning, cognitive flexibility, abstract thinking, rule acquisition, initiating appropriate actions and inhibiting inappropriate actions, and selecting relevant sensory information. Motivation, thinking ahead and considering consequences, initiating plans and changing plans, monitoring and changing behaviors, and planning future behavior are aspects of human behavior that facilitate formation of social networks as well. Without the executive or "overseer" of other brain functions, actions undertaken would likely occur in response to emotions and immediate needs or wants. Impulse control would be lacking because there would be no consideration of the consequence of a particular behavior prior to demonstrating it. For example, a newborn does not have executive functioning skills and thus is impulsive and responds to its own needs. During development of the nervous system in children, the frontal lobes continue to mature well into adolescence and young adulthood, and with it better impulse control and judgment develop as part of the normal developmental process.

One method of assessing executive function is to evaluate working memory. Working memory refers to structures and processes in the brain that allow you to temporarily store and manipulate information. The ability to hold information in this way is a necessary part of being able to utilize the various executive functions described above. It is theorized to differ from short-term memory, which, strictly speaking, is the short-term storage of information. This short-term storage is utilized by the working memory system.

8. How does the brain regulate executive functioning?

Figure 4 illustrates the brain and the location of the frontal lobes that are responsible for executive functioning. Executive functioning is believed to be mediated by the neurotransmitter, dopamine. The brain uses various neurotransmitters such as **serotonin**, norepinephrine, GABA, glutamate, and others for different functions. However, both norepinephrine and dopamine are present in large quantities in the frontal cortex.

Midbrain

The part of the brainstem that is responsible for basic, unconscious body functions.

Working memory

A system in the brain for temporarily storing and managing information required to carry out complex cognitive tasks.

Prefrontal lobe

The anterior part of the cerebral cortex that is implicated in planning complex cognitive actions.

Cerebral cortex

The outer portion of the brain, which is comprised of gray matter and made up of numerous folds that greatly increase the surface area of the brain. Advanced motor function, social abilities, language, and problem solving are coordinated in this area of the brain.

The Basics

Serotonin

A neurotransmitter found in the brain and throughout the body. Serotonin is involved in mood regulation, anxiety, pain perception, appetite, sleep, sexual behavior, and impulsive behavior.

Anterior cingulate gyrus

A part of the limbic system of the brain that is involved in emotional formation and processing, learning, and memory.

Basal ganglia

A region of the brain consisting of three groups of nerve cells (called the caudate nucleus, putamen, and globus pallidus) that are collectively responsible for control of movement.

Parietal lobe

A lobe in the brain that integrates sensory information from different modalities from various parts of the body.

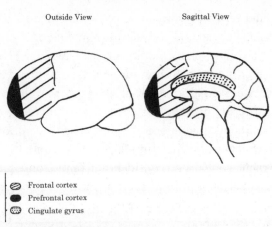

Outside View   Sagittal View

⊘ Frontal cortex
● Prefrontal cortex
⊞ Cingulate gyrus

Figure 4 The brain and the location of the frontal lobes that are responsible for executive functioning.

Different areas of the brain communicate to regulate various components of the attentional system. Executive control is mediated by sections of the brain called the **anterior cingulate gyrus** and the **basal ganglia**; alerting and vigilance are mediated by the right frontal lobe; and selective attention is mediated by the **parietal lobes**, **thalamus**, and midbrain.

The different sections of the brain communicate with the frontal lobe via various neuronal pathways. The frontal lobe system "oversees" the functioning of the rest of the brain, essentially monitoring its own performance so that it can regulate behavior, although entirely how this is done continues to be the subject of research. The specific behavior and cognitive problems that occur due to deficits in the frontal lobe are known from observation and study of patients with frontal lobe damage.

Individuals with frontal lobe damage can exhibit any of the following difficulties:

Cognitive deficits
- Short attention span
- Poor working memory

- Poor short term memory
- Difficulty in planning and reasoning

Behavioral deficits

- Inappropriate aggression
- Inappropriate sexual behavior
- Inappropriate humor
- **Utilization behavior**

Emotional deficits

- Difficulty inhibiting emotions like anger, sadness, etc.
- Depression
- Difficulty understanding others' point of view

Because known frontal lobe damage can cause a variety of symptoms, abberations on a neurochemical level would be expected to result in similar difficulties. While it is recognized that executive function deficits occur secondary to frontal lobe deficits, the specific means by which the frontal lobe controls these aspects of human behavior is an area of ongoing research.

9. What is the DSM-IV-TR?

The *DSM-IV-TR (Diagnostic and Statistical Manual of Mental Disorders, Fourth Edition, Text-Revised)* is considered the standard diagnostic manual for establishing the diagnosis of various mental disorders. Of note, in its introduction, a few caveats are outlined. First, the term mental disorder implies a distinction from physical disorders that is a relic of mind/body dualism. Second, "'mental disorder' lacks a consistent operational definition that covers all situations." Third, the categorical approach has limitations in that discrete entities are assumed when in fact there are no absolute boundaries dividing one disorder from another. Fourth, the criteria for each disorder serve as guidelines only and should not be applied in either a "cookbook" fashion or in an "excessively flexible" manner. Finally, the purpose of the manual is primarily to enhance agreement among clinicians and investigators and is not to imply that any "condition meets legal or other non-medical

Thalamus

A region in the brain that has multiple functions including the relay of information to the cerebral cortex and regulating arousal, awareness, and activity.

Utilization behavior

A condition in which a person has difficulty resisting the impulse to pick up or manipulate objects within his or her visual field or reach.

The Basics

criteria for what constitutes mental disease, mental disorder, or mental disability" (see Introduction and Cautionary Statement of *DSM-IV-TR*).

Treatment plan

The plan agreed on by patient and clinician that will be implemented to treat a mental illness. It incorporates all modalities (therapy and medication).

Only time and the guidance of a skilled clinician who is probing and comprehensive in his or her questioning will help to establish a diagnosis that leads to an effective treatment plan.

It is critical to keep these caveats in mind because it is easy to get caught in a physician's diagnosis, believing that it is set in stone, which it is not. As new information is acquired in treatment, the diagnosis and **treatment plan** may change. Additionally, because of the previously mentioned caveats, it is not uncommon for clinicians to disagree on the diagnosis. When reading the various criteria individually, it is easy to identify with many of them and jump to the conclusion that one has the described condition. Only time and the guidance of a skilled clinician who is probing and comprehensive in his or her questioning will help to establish a diagnosis that leads to an effective treatment plan. The ability to establish a diagnosis is important in developing a treatment plan that restores one's health, and if the treatment plan fails, the first order of business is to reconsider the diagnosis.

10. What is the difference between the fields of psychiatry and psychology?

Historically, the sciences were considered a part of philosophy called natural philosophy because they pertained to thinkers concerned with the state of nature. Psychology was that part of natural philosophy associated with human nature. As philosophers of human nature were primarily concerned with right and wrong, psychology was considered a moral science. This was the purview of philosophers who were contemplating the normal range of human behavior. Alternatively, abnormal behavior, more commonly known as psychopathology, was generally the purview of physicians. Those physicians consisted of either neurologists or general practitioners whose responsibilities included the general medical care of patients committed to asylums for the mentally ill. There was no special training in the diagnosis and treatment of mental illness. Expertise was therefore derived primarily from exposure to those types of patients and not by any specialized training. When science separated from philosophy with the introduction of the experimental method, the field of psychology also began to adopt an equally experimental approach. Psychology retained its status in the university as an academic discipline devoted to understanding how human behavior and the mind worked.

Freud, trained as a neurologist, was the first physician to develop and describe a method of therapy whereby the patient said whatever came to mind, called **free association**. The therapist would listen critically and link up various dreams, memories, and stories the patient related to him and provide an interpretation for the patient as to the unconscious meanings of the patient's narrative. Through these interpretations the patient developed insight, allowing the patient to make changes in both his/her attitudes and behavior so that he/she could be relieved of pain and suffering. Freud coined this method psychoanalysis. This was the beginning of modern psychotherapy. Freud was instrumental in expanding the treatment of mental illness in such a way as to take it out of the asylums and put it into the office. He also strongly believed that, although psychoanalysis required very specialized training, a medical degree was not required in order to learn and practice the technique. Thus, the door was opened to psychologists becoming clinicians rather than solely scientists and philosophers. Since that time, universities and professional schools of psychology have expanded to train psychologists to become clinicians. Psychology students can choose a career track in either research or the practice of clinical psychology. A clinical psychologist typically has undergone four years of undergraduate education and four years of graduate education in psychology, followed by a one-year internship in a mental health care setting, treating patients under the supervision of a senior psychologist.

Psychiatrists have a radically different educational path, having grown as a specialty out of the asylum system where physicians took responsibility for the general health care of the

The Basics

Free association

The mental process of saying aloud whatever comes to mind, suppressing the natural tendency to censor or filter thoughts. This is a technique used in psychoanalysis and in psychodynamic psychotherapy.

mentally ill who were confined to asylums. While psychology has roots in philosophy and thus a similar start in the training, psychiatrists begin studies in human anatomy and physiology as medical students. Graduating with a medical degree and the same educational background as all physicians, psychiatrists spend a year in an internship that may include psychiatry, but must include medicine or some other primary care rotation and neurology. Following internship is the completion of an additional three years as a resident physician, treating patients in a variety of settings under the supervision of a senior psychiatrist. As physicians, psychiatrists are licensed to prescribe medications just as all physicians are. However, because of their specialty they develop a singular expertise in using medications to treat mental illness.

PART TWO

Diagnosis

What are the symptoms of ADHD?

How is ADHD diagnosed?

What are the equivalent adult symptoms
in comparison to the childhood symptoms in the
DSM-IV-TR?

More . . .

11. What are the symptoms of ADHD?

Many people can experience symptoms of ADHD at different times, and you may even wonder, when searching frantically for your keys or forgetting important information, if ADHD is the root of your problems. ADHD symptoms are not episodic or transient however. Key to its diagnosis is that the symptoms are excessive, pervasive, and long-term. That being said, the triad of symptoms of inattention, impulsivity, and hyperactivity characterizes ADHD. Problems with attention can include:

ADHD symptoms are not episodic or transient. Key to its diagnosis is that the symptoms are excessive, pervasive, and long-term.

- Forgetfulness
- Disorganization
- Poor time management
- Frequent misplacing or loss of items
- Frequent tardiness
- Mind wandering during meetings, lectures, or conversations
- Lack of planning

Problems with impulse control and hyperactivity are often manifested in adults by:

- Impatience
- Tendency to interrupt others
- Easy loss of temper
- Low frustration tolerance
- Risk-taking behaviors

The following problems are often associated with ADHD, possibly stemming from the symptoms, or due to problems adjusting to the symptoms:

- Chronic lateness and forgetfulness
- Anxiety
- Low self-esteem

- Employment problems
- Difficulty controlling anger
- Impulsiveness
- Substance abuse or addiction
- Poor organization skills
- Procrastination
- Low frustration tolerance
- Chronic boredom
- Difficulty concentrating when reading
- Mood swings
- Depression
- Relationship problems

Symptoms can vary from one individual to the next. Some individuals are outgoing and social while others can be withdrawn and antisocial. Some people can focus when really interested in something, whereas others cannot under any circumstance. Adults with ADHD may have had school-related difficulties when younger, such as underachieving, frequent disciplinary action, repetition of grades, or history of dropping out. Work-related difficulties are manifest in frequent job changes, wanted or not wanted, and poor performance or lack of job advancement. Socially, symptoms include relationship problems, lower socioeconomic status, illegal substance use, nicotine use, and frequent driving violations.

Liza Miller comments,

I have difficulty with my schoolwork. With treatment, I take time to do my work right rather than half-way. I use flash cards for all subjects that require memorization. I lose things. I lose important items that are both costly and difficult to replace. It is very frustrating and upsetting to lose "my favorite things," and I am not in the financial position to replace them. I don't replace items easily and do not make financial sacrifices. I buy cheaper replacements if the item is necessary.

12. How is ADHD diagnosed?

ADHD is diagnosed as part of a complete psychiatric or other mental health evaluation. It is strictly a clinical diagnosis based upon the clinical history and current symptoms. A clinical history is obtained as part of the evaluation and includes a review of current and past symptoms, psychiatric and medical history, family history, social history, and substance use history. In addition, an assessment of the current **mental status** is included. While there are no tests or procedures to diagnose ADHD, in certain circumstances tests may be ordered in addition to a request for physical examination, in order to rule out any general medical conditions as causes for the symptoms. Depending on the circumstances, the clinician may want to obtain collateral information from family members. School report cards may be requested, and even an interview with the patient's parents may be needed if childhood symptoms are unclear. A developmental history is useful to determine if other problems or conditions existed that are consistent with or suggestive of ADHD. Again, this information may not be known to many adults, but can often be learned from their parents. Based upon the symptoms, history, and mental status, a specific diagnosis can be made. *The Diagnostic and Statistical Manual of Mental Disorders –Fourth Edition-Text Revised (DSM-IV-TR)* (American Psychiatric Association, 2000) defines ADHD by the following symptoms, with criteria needing to be met for either symptoms of inattention, symptoms of hyperactivity-impulsivity, or symptoms of both:

1. Inattention
   - Often fails to give close attention to details or makes careless mistakes in schoolwork, work, or other activities
   - Often has difficulty sustaining attention in tasks or play activities
   - Often does not seem to listen when spoken to directly
   - Often does not follow through on instructions and fails to finish schoolwork, chores, or duties in the workplace

Mental status

A snapshot portrait of one's cognitive and emotional functioning at a particular point in time. It is always included as part of a psychiatric examination.

- Often has difficulty organizing tasks and activities
- Often avoids, dislikes, or is reluctant to engage in tasks that require sustained mental effort
- Often loses things necessary for tasks or activities
- Often easily distracted by extraneous stimuli
- Often forgetful in daily activities

2. Hyperactivity-Impulsivity
- Often fidgets with hands or feet or squirms in seat
- Often leaves seat in classroom or in other situations in which remaining seated is expected
- Often runs about or climbs excessively in situations in which it is inappropriate (in adolescents or adults may be limited to subjective feelings of restlessness)
- Often has difficulty playing or engaging in leisure activities quietly
- Often "on the go" or often acts as if "driven by a motor"
- Often talks excessively
- Often blurts out answers before questions have been completed
- Often has difficulty awaiting turn
- Often interrupts or intrudes on others

Note that at least six symptoms from one or both categories need to have been present for at least six months or more and result in significant impairment in social, academic, or occupational functioning. Such symptoms are also to be present in two or more settings. In addition, such symptoms are to have been present since before the age of seven years. This last point is somewhat controversial in the diagnosis of adult ADHD and is discussed further in Question 20. As with all conditions in the *DSM-IV-TR*, the symptoms also cannot be better accounted for by another condition. This is why a complete evaluation also includes assessment for other disorders that can present with similar complaints. It is particularly important as well that other conditions are screened for, due to the high comorbidity that adults with ADHD have with other disorders.

GERMANTOWN COMMUNITY LIBRARY
GERMANTOWN. WI 53022

Neuropsychological testing is not in and of itself a diagnostic tool for ADHD and is not a required part of the assessment process. It can, however, be useful for clarifying which executive functioning deficits are present and what current functional strengths are present, and can be helpful in identifying areas that need improvement. It is also helpful in revealing and understanding suspected comorbid learning disabilities, such as **dyslexia**.

Dyslexia

A reading disability that alters the way the brain processes written material; such a disability is neurological in origin.

The type of ADHD is also indicated, based upon number of symptoms from each of the previously listed categories. If symptoms from both categories are predominant, it is called ADHD, combined type. If symptoms are predominantly from the inattentive category, the diagnosis is ADHD, predominantly inattentive type; if from the hyperactive-impulsive category, it is ADHD, predominantly hyperactive-impulsive type. The most common type of ADHD diagnosis is ADHD, combined type, which means that there are symptoms present from both categories. There is also a diagnosis called ADHD not otherwise specified, if symptoms are present that do not meet the full criteria (see Question 20).

13. What are the equivalent adult symptoms in comparison to the childhood symptoms in the DSM-IV-TR?

One of the difficulties in diagnosis of ADHD in the adult is that the symptoms listed in the *DSM-IV-TR* do not rigorously match up with adulthood presentations—i.e., adults do not climb furniture and don't typically have difficulty sitting quietly. Hyperactivity in adults usually presents as an inner subjective feeling of restlessness, or some adults pace a lot. Impulsivity presents as mood volatility and temper outbursts, as well as the tendency to interrupt others. Inattentiveness may present as tuning out during conversations, being unable to attend to mundane tasks such as bill paying, and losing and forgetting things.

GERMANTOWN COMMUNITY LIBRARY
GERMANTOWN, WI 53022

Adults, more often than children and adolescents, will have insight into their specific difficulties and seek treatment on their own. Children and adolescents are brought into treatment by a parent or guardian and often do not recognize their specific problems. Also common in adults is that many symptoms are masked by use of compensatory strategies that have been learned over a lifetime of living with ADHD. For example, "forgetfulness" may not be reported as a problem because of diligent use of a planner or personal digital assistant. Hence, the compensatory mechanisms in daily use by adults need to be assessed in order to accurately ascertain symptoms and functioning.

14. Are there any blood tests or other tests for ADHD?

No objective tests, such as blood tests, are available to diagnose ADHD. Your doctor may order blood tests to check for any underlying conditions that may result in similar cognitive symptoms. Blood tests or electrocardiograms may be ordered for baseline purposes, depending on the medication that is to be prescribed because some medications may have effects on certain organ systems in the body. Research protocols look at brain function via various types of brain scans, but these have no utility in clinical practice.

No objective tests, such as blood tests, are available to diagnose ADHD.

While not a required part of an evaluation, various rating scales and self-report forms can be helpful in the evaluation process because they are useful in tracking the progression of the ADHD symptoms over the course of treatment in a quantifiable way. Some clinicians utilize comprehensive diagnostic assessment tools that guide the evaluator in going through a differential diagnostic process, in order to rule out other causes for the symptoms before establishing a diagnosis. Such assessment tools are based upon the *DSM-IV-TR* criteria. These scales are mostly used in research to establish reliability in diagnosis and increase the validity of the study.

Some people will undergo neuropsychological testing to determine if they have ADHD. Because ADHD is a clinical diagnosis, such comprehensive testing is not usually necessary and, by themselves, the results are not diagnostic of ADHD. If used in conjunction with a complete diagnostic evaluation by the testing psychologist, an accurate diagnosis of ADHD can be made. Additional information regarding the use of neuropsychological testing is discussed in Questions 23 and 24.

15. Are there medical conditions that could be the cause for my ADHD?

When considering the diagnosis of ADHD, your clinician will also consider other possible causes for similar symptoms, both psychiatric and medical. In the absence of any physical complaints and with a pervasive presentation, it is unlikely that a medical condition would account for core ADHD symptoms. Certainly the new onset of symptoms suggestive of ADHD would be cause for concern of another medical condition being present, and such an onset would rule out the diagnosis of ADHD. Medical or other conditions that may look like ADHD include:

Petit mal

A type of seizure characterized by brief, unpredictable lapses in consciousness; also known as absence seizures.

Hypothyroidism

Decrease in or absence of thyroid hormone, which is secreted by an endocrine gland near the throat and has wide metabolic effects.

- Medications (e.g., allergy medications) can cause side effects such as hyperactivity
- Seizures, specifically the **petit mal** (absence) seizure, can present with a daydreaming appearance
- Sleep problems such as obstructive sleep apnea can be cause for hyperactivity and attention problems during the day
- Vision and hearing deficits may present as attentive problems for children in the classroom
- Learning disabilities
- **Hypothyroidism**
- Anemia
- Lead toxicity
- Autism

Many of these conditions would have presented in childhood, such as lead toxicity or autism. A thorough medical examination can rule out the majority of the conditions, and if any are suspected a further work-up can be obtained. If a sleep problem is suspected as a cause for the daytime symptoms of inattention and/or hyperactivity, an evaluation in a sleep lab by a sleep specialist may be necessary.

16. How do I know if I have ADHD or unrelated problems with memory and focus?

We all have difficulty with memory and attention from time to time. Who hasn't looked around their home for their keys or wallet? Who hasn't forgotten an appointment? Certain life events and **stressors** can make these difficulties even more pronounced, such as parenthood, a new job, death of a loved one, and so on. The key to the symptoms of inattention actually being secondary to ADHD have to do with its persistence and duration. Symptoms need to have been present (though not necessarily identified at that time) since childhood and need to have been persistent throughout life across situations. There is current controversy as to the necessary age of onset currently identified in the *DSM-IV-TR*, with many clinicians believing that the requirement of symptoms prior to age seven is too early a cutoff. Consideration is being given for a later age of onset in the diagnostic criteria, although still within childhood and/or early adolescence. Over time, symptoms can vary in intensity across different situations as well. The use of screening instruments can help determine if your symptoms should be further evaluated. **Table 1** shows the Adult ADHD Self-Report Scale (ASRS) Screener, which was developed in conjunction with the World Health Organization. If you check yes for most of the questions, consider further evaluation by a qualified practitioner to see if you have ADHD.

Diagnosis

Stressors
Environmental influences on the body and mind that can have gradual adverse effects.

The key to the symptoms of inattention actually being secondary to ADHD have to do with its persistence and duration.

Table 1   Adult ADHD Self-Report Scale (ASRS) Screener

Adult Self-Report Scale-V1.1 (ASRS-V1.1) Screener
from WHO Composite International Diagnostic Interview
© World Health Organization

	Date				

	Never	Rarely	Sometimes	Often	Very Often
Check the box that best describes how you have felt and conducted yourself over the past 6 months. Please give the completed questionnaire to your healthcare professional during your next appointment to discuss the results.					
1. How often do you have trouble wrapping up the final details of a project, once the challenging parts have been done?					
2. How often do you have difficulty getting things in order when you have to do a task that requires organization?					
3. How often do you have problems remembering appointments or obligations?					
4. When you have a task that requires a lot of thought, how often do you avoid or delay getting started?					
5. How often do you fidget or squirm with your hands or feet when you have to sit down for a long time?					
6. How often do you feel overly active and compelled to do things, like you were driven by a motor?					

Add the number of checkmarks that appear in the darkly shaded area. Four (4) or more checkmarks indicate that your symptoms may be consistent with Adult ADHD. It may be beneficial for you to talk with your healthcare provider about an evaluation.

The 6-question Adult Self-Report Scale-Version1.1 (ASRS-V1.1) Screener is a subset of the WHO's 18-question Adult ADHD Self-Report Scale-Version1.1 (Adult ASRS-V1.1) Symptom Checklist.

AT28491 PRINTED IN USA. 3000054636 0903500 ASRS-V1.1 Screener COPYRIGHT © 2003 World Health Organization (WHO). Reprinted with permission of WHO. All rights reserved.

Samantha Miller comments,

ADHD is not simply a problem with memory and focus. I can memorize and I can focus. Having ADHD requires me to do "additional work" in my day-to-day activities. Over many years of practice I have learned ways to manage my symptoms, including learning how to manage my attentional abilities. My motivation to be successful in educational and vocational pursuits took time and dedication. Presently, I am engaged in a practice of Mindfulness Meditation. It has taken over a decade to achieve this practice. Even with this I still need to work at being focused in the present.

17. My spouse doesn't think I have ADHD because I can sit at the computer on the Internet for hours at a time.

While poor attention is typically considered a hallmark of ADHD, the attention problems in ADHD can be conceptualized as difficulty in *shifting* attention, so that when involved in something particularly enjoyable, it can be difficult to have attention drawn away from that activity. This might be seen in a person who is engrossed in a television program or a computer activity who does not respond to another's effort to get his or her attention. It appears the person has "no trouble" paying attention to the computer or television, when in fact the **hyperfocus** is also a problem. Hyperfocus is common during interactive or hands-on activities. When doing something enjoyable, there is more of a tendency to persist in the activity even after others would normally move on to other things. In such a state or "zone," a person with ADHD may not recognize the time that is going by and may then neglect other necessary activities. The hyperfocus may serve as a compensatory mechanism for distractibility in order to be able to complete a task; however, it can be troublesome in that it can lead to failure in school, lost work productivity, and relationship problems with family and friends. Deadlines can be missed or appointments forgotten due to losing track of time. This ability to hyperfocus can also be considered a strength because in this state you may be more apt to make creative breakthroughs or discoveries. Your ability to hyperfocus can be useful for long, complex projects. It is often helpful to set up external cues to pull your attention away from an activity when you know there is a time frame to keep.

Samantha comments,

When I first received the diagnosis of ADHD, my husband wasn't convinced. He believed my difficulties were under my control. He would note how I can sit in front of the television for hours engrossed in various programs. Watching television for long periods has served as my "decompression" from a day of high activity. With

Diagnosis

Hyperfocus

Intense mental concentration on or visualization of a narrow subject.

Bipolar disorder

A mental illness
defined by
episodes of mania
or hypomania,
classically alternating
with episodes of
depression.

*Evaluation for
ADHD should
involve an
assessment for
several other
psychiatric
disorders that
can look like
ADHD.*

Prevalence

Ratio of the
frequency of cases
in the population in
a given time period
of a particular event
to the number
of persons in the
population at risk for
the event.

Mania

A condition
characterized by
elevation of mood
(extreme euphoria or
irritability) associated
with racing thoughts,
decreased need for
sleep, hyperactivity,
and poor impulse
control.

*ongoing education, my husband came to understand my behaviors
and looked at them differently. He became less and less judgmental.
It did, however, take both time and his willingness to learn about
ADHD in adults.*

18. Are there other psychiatric conditions that might be confused with ADHD?

Evaluation for ADHD should involve an assessment for several
other psychiatric disorders that can look like ADHD. Many
symptoms of different illnesses are the same. Concentration can
be a problem in depression as well as in ADHD. Restlessness
and difficulty focusing are features of many anxiety disorders.
Rapid speech and impulsivity are seen in **bipolar disorder**. In
children, ADHD-like symptoms are often seen in the presence
of autism or related conditions. Learning disabilities such as
dyslexia may be confused as a problem with attention. Problems
with anger are seen in many psychiatric disorders, including
ADHD. Therefore, it is very important that a thorough psychi-
atric/medical assessment be done, including screens for many
conditions that can look like ADHD. In addition to a condition
that looks like ADHD, you can also have a comorbid condition
that is present along with the ADHD, another reason why a
thorough diagnostic evaluation is important.

19. My wife is moody, impulsive, and quick to anger. Some people think she is bipolar, but she was diagnosed with ADHD. Is there a connection?

Bipolar disorder and ADHD share many symptoms, but have
differing etiologies, heritability, and **prevalence** rates. People
can mistake ADHD symptoms for the manic phase of bipolar
disorder and bipolar symptoms for ADHD. The symptoms of
mania seen in bipolar disorder are:

- Decreased need for sleep*
- Inflated self-esteem (**grandiosity**)
- Rapid and pressured speech*

- Euphoric (or irritable) mood
- Increased activity level*

These symptoms are further delineated by other criteria in the *DSM-IV-TR* that will not be discussed here, but the reader will note that the three symptoms identified by asterisks are symptoms often seen in ADHD, although not necessarily core symptoms as described in the *DSM-IV-TR*. The mood piece can be characteristic as well if you consider that irritability may be characteristic for some people with ADHD. The decreased need for sleep is often due to the hyperactivity and high energy level associated with ADHD and may be experienced as **insomnia**. The difference from bipolar individuals can be subtle in that, during a manic state, the lack of sleep is not experienced as insomnia in which sleep is desired, but is due to adequate energy levels and lack of fatigue. The same goes for activity level, which can have subtle differences based upon the type of mood that is associated with it. Speech in ADHD individuals is often rapid, characterized by a tendency to interrupt, but also with a subtle difference from **pressured speech** characterized by mania. These differences are not always easy to detect. This is where duration and pattern of illness becomes important diagnostically. Bipolar disorder is episodic and has an identifiable onset. ADHD is chronic with an onset in childhood or early adolescence. ADHD symptoms don't go away. A manic or **hypomanic** episode will often cycle to a **euthymic** (baseline) or depressed state. The proper diagnosis is important for treatment considerations. It is also possible to have comorbid ADHD and bipolar disorder, which is discussed in Question 76.

20. I have all the symptoms of ADHD but do not believe my symptoms started until adolescence. Would ADHD be a valid diagnosis?

The *DSM-IV-TR* currently requires an onset of at least some symptoms to occur prior to the age of seven. In some cases, such an onset cannot be corroborated. In others, it is clear that

---

Diagnosis

Grandiosity

The tendency to consider the self or one's ideas better or more superior to what is reality.

Insomnia

A condition marked by the inability to fall asleep, middle of the night awakening, or early morning awakening.

Pressured speech

Characterized by the need to keep speaking; it is difficult to interrupt someone with this type of speech. This is commonly seen in manic or hypomanic mood states.

Hypomania

A milder form of mania with the same symptoms but of lesser intensity.

Euthymic

To be characterized by moderation of mood.

the symptoms did not manifest until adolescence. This age criterion is currently under dispute in the psychiatric community and is under reconsideration for a future revision of the *DSM*. At present however, it is still possible to have a diagnosis of ADHD without having met the age requirement. There is a diagnostic category called Attention-Deficit/Hyperactivity Disorder not otherwise specified, or ADHD NOS. The *DSM-IV-TR* states that this diagnosis "is for disorders with prominent symptoms of inattention or hyperactivity/impulsivity that do not meet criteria for Attention-Deficit/Hyperactivity Disorder." The *DSM-IV-TR* also cites two examples that would meet this definition:

- Late-onset ADHD for which the patient meets all criteria except the onset prior to age 7
- Subthreshold ADHD for which the patient does not meet full symptom criteria but is significantly impaired by ADHD symptoms

In terms of assessing the validity of the age criteria, studies have examined patients with an early age of onset and late age of onset of ADHD, and have found that they do not differ in symptom severity, type of impairment, or in persistence of the disorder. One study has found that the age criteria have actually reduced the accuracy of identifying impaired cases of ADHD. The treatment of ADHD NOS is the same as the other types.

21. I've been diagnosed with ADHD. What do I tell my family and friends?

Although of late there is greater understanding in our society of various psychiatric conditions many people deal with, such as depression, anxiety and ADHD, there is still a reluctance to reveal such difficulties to others for fear of stigma or shame. Myths about ADHD, such as its being a problem with "laziness" persist and can remain in the subconscious regardless of the understanding you have obtained about the disorder. Certainly it can be a relief to inform close family and friends who may have recognized over the time you have known each other that you have trouble with being on time, remembering appointments, becoming easily frustrated, and so on. Perhaps friends and/or family members have teased you over the years because of your difficulties. Providing them with information that you have ADHD and then educating them about the condition can ease some of the long-standing misconceptions that have been held about you as a person. Perhaps their understanding can help alleviate any shame or guilt you have experienced or improve your self-esteem when you can accept that you have a condition through no fault of your own.

Ultimately, however, you have to decide who really needs to know and who does not. As with any medical condition, what you receive treatment for is really a private matter, and discretion should be used regarding the sharing of information. One setting in which it would be prudent not to share this information is the college setting, as stimulant diversion is a common practice on college campuses. If friends and acquaintances know you have stimulant medication, there is a good possibility you will be asked to provide someone with "just one pill" to help them out. Even if you recognize the risks of letting others use your medication, it can be a hassle to have others asking you for it. Therefore, it is best if no one knows you have the medication to begin with.

Samantha comments,

I was very open about it and continue to be. Identifying and recognizing relationship problems as due to ADHD actually helped my relationships. Family and friends can better understand why it is I do what I do and can help me stay on track. I've never considered my ADHD to be something I need to hide.

22. Is ADHD a type of learning disability?

Although a common misperception, ADHD is not considered a learning disability. The reason for the misperception is probably that ADHD can affect learning and often has

The definition of a learning disability is to have a deficit in a specific skill area while performing at a higher level intellectually.

learning disabilities associated with it. The definition of a learning disability is to have a deficit in a specific skill area while performing at a higher level intellectually. The diagnosis is made when there is a significant discrepancy between IQ and performance on achievement tests. A person with a reading disability would be expected to perform fine in math unless there was a specific disability in that subject as well. In contrast, ADHD affects learning across all subject areas, not just one. About 30% to 40% of individuals with ADHD have comorbid learning disabilities, so it is important to screen for them and to conduct further testing when indicated.

While ADHD is not a learning disability, it can be classified as a disability under the Individuals with Disabilities Education Act (IDEA) in order to determine eligibility for special education services. Students may be eligible under the categories of specific learning disability, other health impairment, or emotional disturbance. If criteria are not met under the IDEA, another option for obtaining services in the school setting is found under Section 504 of the Rehabilitation Act. This section has different eligibility criteria for receiving services without being in need of special education services.

23. How does neuropsychological testing differ from psychological testing?

Both types of testing are performed by psychologists and consist of a series of paper-and-pencil tests along with history and review of symptoms. Neuropsychological testing is more comprehensive than psychological testing and its providers have received additional training in administration of the testing and interpretation of the results.

Psychological testing

The use of samples of behavior to infer generalizations about a given individual.

Psychological testing is utilized to provide information about a patient's personality and emotional functioning. This may be needed to aid in the differential diagnosis of behavioral or psychiatric conditions when the patient's history and symptomatology are not readily attributable to a particular psychiatric diagnosis and the questions to be answered by psychological testing could not be resolved by a psychiatric/diagnostic interview. Such testing is also often completed as part of the assessment process in certain mental health or substance abuse facilities and may be needed to develop treatment recommendations after various medications or therapeutic interventions have resulted in treatment failure. Psychological tests include self-report questionnaires and rating scales, projective tests (e.g., Rorschach, Thematic Aperception Test), and cognitive testing (e.g., tests for intellectual functioning or IQ and academic achievement tests).

Neuropsychological testing is more comprehensive and typically includes elements of psychological testing, but it also uses additional tests that measure and identify cognitive impairment and functioning in individuals. Specific cognitive functions that are evaluated include:

- Short-term and long-term memory
- The ability to learn new skills and solve problems
- Attention, concentration, and distractibility
- Logical and abstract reasoning functions
- The ability to understand and express language
- Visual-spatial organization
- Visual-motor coordination
- Planning, synthesizing, and organizing abilities

Neuropsychological testing is obtained when children don't achieve appropriate developmental milestones, in head injured patients, in patients with Parkinson's disease or other neurological diseases, in stroke patients, and in dementia patients.

A clinical diagnosis, ADHD is not diagnosed by neuropsychological testing, although results on such testing can be highly supportive of such a diagnosis. Such testing may be desirable when the diagnosis of ADHD is unclear, if treatment has failed, or in the presence of suspected learning disabilities. Such testing is also typically required when accommodations

Neuropsychological testing

The assessment of brain functioning through structured and systematic behavioral observation.

Diagnosis

are being requested for school or standardized tests. Having a diagnosis of ADHD does not automatically allow for the attainment of such accommodations, as functional impairments need to be demonstrated for the purposes of academic work or test taking. Formalized testing documents the specific impairments and how the accommodations would be helpful. Depending upon the findings, various interventions for within the school or work environments can be suggested to help with the symptoms.

24. What is the role of neuropsychological testing in diagnosing adult ADHD?

The diagnosis of adult ADHD is based upon the clinical assessment and history. Neuropsychological testing can be helpful in evaluating symptoms when the diagnosis is unclear, when there is substantial comorbidity, when learning disabilities are suspected, or even when it is difficult to establish whether symptoms began in childhood. The results of the testing need to be considered in the context of the clinical presentation and history of the patient and should not be used alone for diagnosis. Tests that may be performed as part of a neuropsychological assessment in adults include:

- Continuous performance testing, which evaluates selective and sustained attention
- Digit symbol and coding tests, which evaluate perceptual-motor speed
- Digit span tests, which evaluate working memory
- Stroop-Color Word Test, which evaluates verbal learning and response inhibition
- Wisconsin Card Sorting Test, which evaluates visual skills and working memory
- Trail-Making Test, which evaluates visual-motor speed and task-switching skills
- Wechsler Adult Intelligence Scale, which evaluates intellectual functioning

- Verbal fluency, which evaluates fluency of verbal productivity

Research has demonstrated that adults with ADHD perform more poorly than controls in various neuropsychological tests; however, studies have not shown a connection between test results and the presence of functional impairment, which is a requirement for a diagnosis of ADHD. Deficits found on various neuropsychological tests are found in frontal lobe dysfunction in general, which means that the clinical presentation and history must be part of the assessment for ADHD. Results of neuropsychological testing can be used for requesting accommodations in academic settings, and are a requirement for such for standardized examinations, but keep in mind that insurance companies may not provide reimbursement for neuropsychological testing when performed for assessment of ADHD and academic needs.

25. I've had difficulty concentrating at school and tried a stimulant. I was able to get a lot of work done. Does this mean I have ADHD?

Stimulants will improve the concentration and focus in anyone who takes them, but if not prescribed for a legitimate condition, they are actually being misused. If you have concerns regarding your concentration abilities and are concerned about the possibility of ADHD, then you should obtain a thorough evaluation to determine the cause of your symptoms. Concentration can be adversely affected by many psychiatric and medical conditions, and a beneficial effect from a stimulant is not diagnostic of ADHD. As a controlled substance with potential for addiction, use of a stimulant in a way that was not prescribed can easily lead to continued misuse and abuse. This is an issue of concern in many colleges because it appears to be a safe way to stay alert and focused when faced with an abundance of work. The use of stimulants in this way, however, can be dangerous. Without a proper evaluation you do not know what, if any, medication is warranted, whether the dosage is appropriate for you specifically, and whether or not contraindications exist for your taking a stimulant or other medication, many of which can put your health at significant risk. If you have a concern regarding your concentration abilities, it is prudent to meet with your doctor to be evaluated and determine the best course of action.

26. Who is qualified to diagnose and treat ADHD?

Many clinicians of various educational backgrounds are qualified to diagnose and treat ADHD. Physicians who can diagnose and treat ADHD include psychiatrists, neurologists, internists, and pediatricians. Internists and pediatricians, however, may choose to refer you to a mental health provider depending upon their comfort level in treating ADHD. Because ADHD has been commonly considered a disorder of childhood, more pediatricians than adult medical practitioners are adept at its treatment. Of the different physicians, a psychiatrist may also be able to provide psychotherapy in addition to the medication management. Psychiatric nurse practitioners are skilled in the diagnosis and treatment of ADHD and are also able to prescribe medication. Because ADHD has been relatively recently recognized as a common disorder in adulthood, it is worthwhile to seek a psychiatrist or nurse practitioner who is comfortable and experienced in its treatment. Child and adolescent psychiatrists typically work with adults as well, and they are usually experienced in treatment of ADHD across the lifespan. Other mental health practitioners such as psychologists and clinical social workers can diagnose ADHD, but may need to refer you to a psychiatrist for a medical assessment and treatment recommendations. Most insurance plans have participants who can provide mental health services, although the choices available on a given plan are sometimes limited. Geographic location also may dictate your choice of practitioner because there are shortages of certain clinicians in some areas of the United

States (e.g., child and adolescent psychiatrists). For adjunctive treatment to medication, many mental health practitioners can provide various types of psychotherapy to address either ADHD symptoms or comorbid conditions. These practitioners include:

- Social workers
- Psychologists
- Psychiatric nurse specialists
- Psychiatrists

In seeking a mental health specialist, it is important to choose someone with proper credentials and training. Anyone can call himself or herself a psychotherapist without having specialized training or a degree. It is appropriate to ask the therapist about his or her training and background in the assessment and treatment of ADHD. Credentials for the noted mental health specialists follow.

Social workers provide a full range of mental health services, including assessment, diagnosis, and treatment. They have completed undergraduate work in social work or other fields, followed by post-graduate education to obtain a Master's of Social Work (MSW) or a doctorate degree. An MSW is required in order to practice as a clinical social worker or to provide therapy. Most states require practicing social workers to be licensed, certified, or registered. Post-graduate education is two years with courses in social welfare, psychology, family systems, child development, diagnosis, and child and elder abuse/neglect. During the two years of coursework, social work students participate in internships concordant with their interest. Following completion of the Master's program, direct clinical supervision for a period of time, which may vary from state to state, is usually required before applying for a license.

Psychologists have completed undergraduate work, followed by several years of post-graduate studies, in order to receive

In seeking a mental health specialist, it is important to choose someone with proper credentials and training.

a doctorate degree (PhD or PsyD) in psychology. Graduate psychology education includes study of a variety of subjects, notably statistics, social psychology, developmental psychology, personality theory, psychological testing (paper and pencil tests to help assess personality characteristics, intelligence, learning difficulties, and evidence of psychopathology), psychotherapeutic techniques, history and philosophy of psychology, and psychopharmacology and **physiological** psychology. Following the coursework, a year is spent in a mental health setting providing psychotherapeutic care and psychological testing under the supervision of a senior psychologist. Psychologists must demonstrate a minimum number of hours (usually around 1,500) before they are eligible to sit for state psychology licensure exams.

Psychiatric nurse specialists have completed undergraduate work, typically in nursing, and obtained post-graduate education in nursing at the master's or doctorate level. Master's programs are two years with coursework consisting of study in physiology, pathophysiology, psychopathology, pharmacology, **psychosocial** and psychotherapeutic treatment modalities, advanced nursing, and diagnosis. The training includes clinical work under supervision. Licensing varies from state to state.

Psychiatrists are medical doctors with specialized training in psychiatry. They have completed undergraduate work followed by four years of medical school. Medical education is grounded in basic sciences of anatomy, physiology, pharmacology, microbiology, histology, immunology, and pathology, followed by two years of clinical rotations through specialties that include medicine, surgery, pediatrics, obstetrics and gynecology, family practice, and psychiatry (as well as other elective clerkships). During this time, medical students must pass two examinations toward licensure. After graduation from medical school, physicians have a year of internship that includes at least four months in a primary care specialty such as medicine or pediatrics and two months of neurology. Following internship, physicians must take and pass a third

Physiological

Pertaining to functions and activities of the living matter, such as organs, tissues, or cells.

Psychosocial

Pertaining to environmental circumstances that can impact one's psychological well-being.

exam toward licensure in order to be eligible for licensure (and subsequently practice) in any state. Psychiatrists-in-training have three more years of specialty training in residency, the successful completion of which makes them eligible for board certification. Following residency, many psychiatrists pursue further training in fellowships that can last an additional two years. Such fellowships include child and adolescent psychiatry, geriatric psychiatry, consultation-liaison psychiatry, addiction psychiatry, forensic psychiatry, and research. To become board certified, psychiatrists take both written and oral examinations. Certain psychiatry specialties also have a board certification process. Board certification is not a requirement to practice and may not be obtained immediately upon completion of residency, although many hospitals and insurance companies do require physicians to be board certified within a specified number of years in order to treat patients.

In addition to seeking a private practitioner for mental health services, there are different types of facilities/programs where you may obtain an evaluation and treatment, in which various mental health specialists work, including community mental health centers, hospital psychiatry departments and outpatient clinics, university-affiliated programs, social service agencies, and employee assistance programs.

Diagnosis

PART THREE

Risk, Prevention, and Epidemiology

What causes ADHD?

I have recently been diagnosed with ADHD. What are the risks my children will inherit it?

What are the risks of untreated ADHD?

More . . .

27. What causes ADHD?

The exact cause of ADHD is not known and there are likely several causes. What is known is that ADHD is a highly heritable disorder that runs in families, and various genes studied thus far are suspected to be involved. Neuroimaging has shown a link between ADHD and brain structure, brain neurochemistry, and functional brain differences in areas of attention and impulse control. Genetics do not, however, cover the whole picture because twin studies do not show 100% **concordance** rates in identical twins. Since identical twins share all the same genes, any condition that was completely genetic would be seen in both twins. What would influence the subsequent development of ADHD in a person with genetic vulnerability is not known. There are, however, additional environmental factors that can cause ADHD in the absence of genetic contribution, as well as possibly facilitate its development in someone with a genetic predisposition. These are:

Concordance

In genetics, a similarity in a twin pair with respect to presence or absence of illness.

- In-utero exposure to nicotine and/or drugs
- Lead poisoning
- Extremely low birth weight
- Head trauma
- Oxygen deprivation at birth

Smoking during pregnancy is one of the most studied and consistently identified prenatal risk factors for later development of ADHD. This risk can be independent of a genetic link for ADHD, but can also increase risk in the presence of a genetic susceptibility. What should be noted is that an insult that can affect the neurodevelopment of the fetal or perinatal brain can result in ADHD.

28. I have recently been diagnosed with ADHD. What are the risks my children will inherit it?

ADHD is a highly heritable disorder with a heritability rate of 0.75. To put that into perspective, the heritability rate is similar for both schizophrenia and bipolar disorder, while the heritability rate of major depression is lower, at about 0.40. A person's height has a heritability rate of close to 0.90 and eye color inheritance has a rate of 0.98. Evidence for the heritability of ADHD includes:

- Concordance rates for ADHD in twin studies are ~80% for identical twins while concordance rates in nonidentical twins are ~30%.
- In **adoption studies**, rates of ADHD are higher in biological relatives than in adoptive relatives.
- Over 25% of **first-degree relatives** of children with ADHD have ADHD, in contrast to 5% in control groups.
- Parents and siblings of children with ADHD are 2 to 8 times more likely to develop ADHD than the general population.

Adoption study

A scientific study designed to control for genetic relatedness and environmental influences by comparing siblings adopted into different families.

First-degree relative

Immediate biologically related family member, such as biological parents or full siblings.

Keep in mind that while the genetic risk is high, the severity level of symptoms may be different. Efforts to reduce any prenatal factors that can increase risk for ADHD might be partaken if pregnant, but other than that there is no evidence for a means of reducing the risk that your child will develop ADHD. What can be helpful is early recognition if symptoms become apparent in order to determine the best intervention for your child.

Keep in mind that while the genetic risk is high, the severity level of symptoms may be different.

Samantha comments,

To my knowledge there is a very strong risk. The genetic data suggests that ADHD is the most heritable of all psychiatric conditions. The professional (also a colleague of mine) who diagnosed my daughter (in her teen years) had already recognized it in me. When I brought my daughter to her for a consultation it was necessary to describe in great detail my daughter's behavior. It was then that I realized I shared very similar behaviors.

29. Are there specific risk factors associated with getting ADHD?

There are risk factors one can change and risk factors one cannot. You cannot change the genes inherited from your parents, but you can use the knowledge of your family history to help make choices in life to reduce other risk factors contributing to the probability of developing a particular disease. For many psychiatric disorders, the genetic risk is present but also considered heavily influenced by environmental factors. This is true for many psychiatric disorders, but less so for ADHD. With its high heritability rate, there is less of a role of environment in terms of risk, and certainly by adulthood, you either have it or do not, but it is useful to know some of the connections as well as real environmental risks that can be changed. Some of the associations are:

- Gender: In children the male to female ratio is 4:1, but it becomes closer to 1:1 by adulthood.
- Age: Age of onset is childhood, although it is thought for some that symptoms develop in adolescence. ADHD would not develop in adulthood.
- Family history: There is a 40% chance one parent will have ADHD if a child has it.
- Low birth weight: Increased risk.
- Lead poisoning: Associated with development of ADHD.
- Prenatal nicotine exposure: Associated with development of ADHD.
- Prenatal drug and/or alcohol exposure: Associated with development of ADHD.
- Psychiatric disorders: Higher rates of ADHD in the presence of depression, bipolar disorder, generalized anxiety disorder, and substance abuse.

In ADHD, the risk factors one has control over are very limited when compared to diseases such as heart disease, which offers opportunities for lowering cholesterol, blood pressure, and weight through various options including diet, exercise, smoking cessation, and prescription medications. It is often difficult, if not impossible, to change exposure to any of the risk factors for ADHD mentioned above, except at the level of prenatal care. Yet the perceived level of control over ADHD symptoms is much greater than for other diseases, with myths that persist in our society regarding the level of control a person has over their ADHD symptoms.

Due to the higher risk for comorbidity associated with ADHD, risk for development of depression or anxiety disorders may be mitigated by the reduction of psychosocial stress as well as treating the ADHD and engaging in psychotherapy or other measures to learn coping skills for living with ADHD.

30. Is ADHD an artifact of American society?

Due to the prevalence of ADHD in the United States, some believe that it is a phenomenon of American society and culture. Another theory, however, is that it is common in races and societies worldwide, but not recognized by the medical community elsewhere. The World Health Organization recognizes the disorder under the grouping of disorders called hyperkinetic disorders, within which there are several types, all of which have hyperactivity associated with them. Data from studies in the 1970s cites a 20-fold greater prevalence of the disorder in the United States as compared to England, but subsequent research that examined the data used in those studies found hyperactivity scores to be similar across studies from different countries, but that differences in definition of the condition of hyperactivity may have accounted for the appearance of a greater prevalence. Subsequent studies also found that rates of hyperactivity are the same between the United States and the United Kingdom, and that different diagnostic practices, rather than differences in behavior of the children, reflect the different interpretations of the disorder. Faraone et al. (2003) reviewed 50 worldwide studies done on ADHD in order to compare prevalence rates. Results showed that while certain populations may have a lower prevalence of ADHD symptoms, prevalence rates were generally at least as high in non–US children as in US children.

31. Is the diagnosis of ADHD increasing?

Recognition of ADHD as a lifelong disorder that does not end in adolescence has resulted in more cases of ADHD being diagnosed in adults. The condition has always been present, however, and the prevalence rate is not believed to be increasing. ADHD is not only under-diagnosed in the adult population, but is missed in children and adolescents as well. Prevalence rates of ADHD in children and adolescents are estimated to be between 5% and 8% with, contrary to popular belief, less than 50% having been diagnosed and even less receiving treatment. Only 25% of adults with ADHD were first recognized to have the disorder in childhood and only about 10% of adults with ADHD are now receiving treatment. Girls have a lower rate of diagnosis than boys; however, the diagnosis becomes equal in adulthood. It is thought that girls are more likely to have the inattentive type of ADHD and thus, due to the absence of disruptive behavior, are not as apt to be recognized as having difficulty during school years. Developmentally, the hyperactive and impulsive symptoms dramatically decline into adulthood, whereas the inattentive symptoms tend to be more stable. It may be that due to the apparent decline of hyperactive and impulsive symptoms, that ADHD was once believed to resolve prior to adulthood.

Many individuals have difficulty taking the first step of making an appointment with a mental health practitioner.

32. A family member has ADHD. Is there anything I can do to help?

Helping your family member seek treatment is one of the more important ways to assist. Many individuals have difficulty taking the first step of making an appointment with a mental health practitioner. If the person is already in treatment, helping him or her remember the appointments and providing encouragement to stay in the treatment will be of tremendous help. Accompanying your family member to any appointments to provide feedback to the clinician can be of help, especially since it can be difficult for individuals with ADHD to recognize all their symptoms. It is particularly helpful if you knew the family member as a child to provide history. If he or she is on medication, assistance and reminders to take medication are useful, as lapses in **compliance** with medication are common. Because many people with ADHD have gaps in their attention, help your family member by making sure he or she has heard everything you've said by having him or her repeat what you've said. By understanding ADHD as an illness, you can also help by not judging and blaming, but by gently pointing out undesirable behaviors. Providing feedback in private without being judgmental can be helpful as well.

33. What are the risks of untreated ADHD?

Risks of untreated ADHD may be looked at from the perspective of both the individual and society. It may be easy for an individual to forgo treatment for ADHD because, on the surface, it can appear that ADHD may cause little, if any, significant impairment in day-to-day living. Potential consequences of untreated ADHD can be quite serious, however, and include:

- Academic limitations
- Low self-esteem
- Increased risk for injuries
- Smoking
- Substance abuse
- Motor vehicle accidents and other moving violations
- Occupational problems
- Legal problems
- Relationship problems

As can be seen from this list, symptoms of ADHD can impact nearly all areas of living and create significant functional

Compliance

Extent that behavior follows medical advice, such as by taking prescribed treatments. Compliance can refer to medications as well as to appointments and psychotherapy sessions.

impairment. With academic limitations, future job prospects are limited, and thus income potential and career growth. Low self-esteem can make you susceptible to depression and even worse functioning. Smoking and substance abuse have their own list of consequences. Motor vehicle accidents are more common in individuals with ADHD and studies have shown reduced moving violations amongst ADHD patients who are on medication. Occupational problems are evidenced by high job turnover due to frequent quitting or due to firings, and relationship problems result in higher divorce rates.

From a societal standpoint, the costs of untreated ADHD are connected to loss of work productivity, direct and indirect medical costs, auto accident-related costs, and incarceration costs. Adults with ADHD tend to be undereducated with fewer graduating high school. If they go on to college, fewer are able to complete their studies, thus affecting their job market viability. With the high risk of unemployment due to job loss as well, household income goes down. Medical costs are higher due to higher worker's compensation claims with studies also showing higher annual medical costs for individuals with ADHD. High rates of comorbid mental health conditions both raise the use of medical services and result in higher costs due to consequences of those disorders. Costs of automobile accidents result in higher insurance premiums for everyone, and the cost of injury is an additional societal burden. Incarceration rates are higher for individuals with ADHD, with studies showing that inmates with ADHD comprise 40% of the population in prison.

34. Is there a link between parenting and development of ADHD?

No link has been shown between development of ADHD and parenting styles, other than the possibility of early childhood abuse contributing to the development of ADHD (secondary to head trauma). Parenting styles can certainly be contributory to certain types of disruptive behavior disorders in children and adolescents, such as oppositional defiant disorder (ODD) or conduct disorder (CD). While the cause of ODD and CD are not known, theories of their origins include the presence of a developmental problem and its being due to a response to negative interactions with the parents. The techniques used by parents and authority figures on some children bring about the oppositional defiant behavior. So in contrast to ADHD, ODD is a psychological condition that is responsive to external situations and circumstances. CD can subsequently develop in ODD children and is considered a more serious behavioral condition. Oppositional defiant disorder occurs at a higher rate in children with ADHD, with about 50% of children with ADHD also developing ODD or CD at some point during their development. The difference between ADHD and ODD or CD is that behavior problems that occur secondary to ADHD are not deliberate or willful. Behavior problems that are secondary to ODD and CD are willful. The risk for ODD or CD in ADHD children may be due to the difficulty in parenting a child with ADHD in that the characteristic impulsivity and hyperactivity facilitates development of conflict in parent-child, teacher-child, and peer relationships. These conflicts can promote the development of defiance and aggression. Parenting styles may need to be modified in response to the child with ADHD and understanding of the child's behavior (i.e., recognizing it is not willful or intended to be hurtful) can go a long way in reducing the stress in parenting a child with ADHD and thus minimizing the risk for worsening difficulties later on. So while parenting behavior is not a cause of ADHD, parenting styles can affect the outcomes of ADHD.

The difference between ADHD and ODD or CD is that behavior problems that occur secondary to ADHD are not deliberate and willful. Behavior problems that are secondary to ODD and CD are willful.

PART FOUR

Treatment

What are the different types of treatment for ADHD?

Does the type of ADHD I have determine the type of treatment I need?

What are the different types of medication used to treat ADHD?

More . . .

35. What are the different types of treatment for ADHD?

The main treatment modalities for ADHD fall under the categories of pharmacological treatments and psychosocial treatments. **Pharmacological** treatments have been in use for decades and have a long track record of high **efficacy** for this disorder. Psychosocial treatments may or may not address the core ADHD symptoms, but can be useful to address coping skills and comorbid conditions. Psychosocial treatments do not bring about remission of ADHD symptoms, as can be the case for certain depressive and anxiety disorders. Rather, these treatments help patients work around their ADHD symptoms.

Pharmacological treatment typically involves the use of stimulant medications, although non-stimulant medications are available for ADHD as well, some of which may include **antidepressant** medication. The benefits and rationale of the different choices of medication are discussed below, but stimulants are very effective and are considered a first line treatment. When additional psychiatric conditions are present, the medication choice may depend in part upon the other condition, and it may mean that more than one medication needs to be taken for each condition.

Psychosocial treatments include various therapeutic modalities, including individual psychotherapy, group therapy, and family or couples therapy. Additional interventions may include coaching (Question 44) and organizational assistance. Because ADHD is a brain disorder, individual psychotherapy alone is typically better suited to addressing life issues affected by the ADHD. In other words, a treatment course of individual therapy would not be expected to resolve attention problems for example. Cognitive behavioral therapy as an individual therapy modality can be useful in teaching techniques to work around the attention deficits present in ADHD. Couples or family therapy can be helpful in addressing the strain upon relationships that ADHD often causes. While not

Pharmacological

Pertaining to all chemicals that, when ingested, cause a physiological process to occur in the body. Psychopharmacologic refers to those physiologic processes that have direct psychological effects.

Efficacy

The capacity to produce a desired effect, such as the performance of a drug or therapy in relieving symptoms of depression such as feeling down, trouble concentrating, etc.

Antidepressant

A drug specifically marketed for and capable of relieving the symptoms of clinical depression. It is often used to treat conditions other than depression.

defined as a therapy, coaching serves to facilitate changes in your life that help work with the ADHD symptoms.

As part of an evaluation, your clinician will consider the most appropriate treatment plan for your ADHD. With no associated comorbidities, medication alone may be recommended. If there are additional concerns such as self-esteem issues, relationship issues, or other disorders, a specialized therapeutic approach may be recommended. **Table 2** outlines the common types of therapy and the focus of each. The type of therapy chosen will also depend upon cost, duration, or patient fit. Typical frequency of therapy sessions is once per week, but may be higher or lower depending upon your individual needs. Other treatments that have not been rigorously studied include **EEG biofeedback** and alternative medications.

EEG biofeedback

A learning strategy that enables persons to alter their brain waves.

Table 2   Common Types of Therapy

Therapy	Duration	Illness/Focus	Theory
Psychoanalytic or psychodynamic	Few months to few years	Personality disorders, coping skills	Unconscious conflicts from childhood
Behavioral	6–20 sessions	Anxiety disorders, depression, psychosomatic symptoms	Symptom reinforcement
Cognitive	10–20 sessions	Depression, obsessive-compulsive disorder	Negative thoughts
Interpersonal	12 sessions	Depression	Relationship focused
Dialectical behavioral	One year or greater	Borderline personality disorder	Reduction of self-injurious behaviors
Psychoeducational	Long-term	Families of schizophrenic patients	Support and education
Supportive	Brief	Acute grief reactions	Reinforcing patient's strengths
Group	Open-ended or time-limited	Mood disorders, anxiety disorders, schizophrenia	Support and education
Family	Short- to long-term	Family roles, support, education, dynamics	Various

36. Does the type of ADHD I have determine the type of treatment I need?

All types of ADHD respond to the same types of treatment. For example, the hyperactive-impulsive subtype of ADHD would be treated in the same way as the inattentive subtype of ADHD.

All types of ADHD respond to the same types of treatment. For example, the hyperactive-impulsive subtype of ADHD would be treated in the same way as the inattentive subtype of ADHD. Choice of medication is not based upon the type of ADHD. However, some of the therapeutic modalities are likely better suited for addressing different aspects of ADHD, with behavioral interventions potentially helpful for impulsivity and organizational problems. Any comorbidity associated with the ADHD could determine the most appropriate treatment intervention. For example, from a pharmacological perspective, the presence of a comorbid tic disorder may warrant a trial of a non-stimulant such as atomoxetine. An associated anxiety or depressive disorder may benefit from a specific type of therapy as noted in Table 2.

Different symptom presentations may affect choice of pharmacotherapy, as the various medications available for treating ADHD have different mechanisms and durations of action. Question 37 describes the various medication choices for ADHD and questions that follow discuss how they might be utilized.

37. What are the different types of medication used to treat ADHD?

There are a few different classes of medications that are used in the treatment of ADHD, although only some stimulants and one nonstimulant are approved for the treatment of ADHD in adults. Most of the medications used affect the noradrenergic system, albeit with different mechanisms of action. Medication choices include many medications within the following classes:

Stimulants
- Amphetamine
- Methylphenidate

Nonstimulants
- Atomoxetine

Antidepressants
- Venlafaxine
- Bupropion
- Tricyclics

Antihypertensives
- Clonidine
- Guanfacine

Wake-promoting agents
- Modafinil

Note that the FDA has approved only some of the available stimulants and one nonstimulant, atomoxetine, for the treatment of adult ADHD. While not all stimulants have been approved for the treatment of ADHD in adults, it is generally expected that all can be helpful. **Table 3** lists the medications approved for adult ADHD thus far, along with the given trade names. Other medications have evidence for their efficacy but have not been presented for review by the FDA for approval.

Table 3   FDA-Approved Medications for Adult ADHD

Generic Name	Trade Name
Methylphenidate	Concerta
Dexmethylphenidate	Focalin XR
Lisdexamfetamine	Vyvanse
Mixed amphetamine salt	Adderall XR
Atomoxetine	Strattera

The first and only nonstimulant approved for the treatment of ADHD is atomoxetine. While the response rate to stimulants is higher, there are many reasons that availability of a nonstimulant medication choice is important. Stimulants are not always well tolerated, with the loss of appetite and sleep difficulties presenting a problem for some people. In addition, stimulants can exacerbate underlying mood or anxiety disorders, exacerbate tics, and be subject to abuse. Cardiovascular risks may be of more concern with stimulants when used in the adult population. In contrast to a stimulant, atomoxetine does not provide an immediate response—it takes between 4 and 6 weeks for its full effects to be apparent (once on the right dose). Therefore, in the absence of any contraindications, it is common practice to try a stimulant first; any positive or negative effects will be ascertained early in the treatment. If ineffective, a switch to atomoxetine is then usually made.

Other medications used in the treatment of adult ADHD include bupropion and venlafaxine, both of which come in extended release formulations. These are both antidepressants that have shown some evidence for efficacy on ADHD symptoms, thought likely due to their dopaminergic and noradrenergic effects. These treatments can be considered in the presence of comorbid depression or anxiety, or if other interventions have not been helpful. Tricyclic antidepressants are norepinephrine and serotonin reuptake inhibitors that have some demonstrated efficacy in ADHD as well, but they have more significant adverse effects, including cardiac effects, that limit their utility. The more commonly prescribed tricyclic antidepressants are imipramine, desipramine, and nortriptyline.

An additional off-label use of medication for ADHD that is commonly used in children is clonidine and guanfacine. Guanfacine does not need to be dosed as frequently as clonidine, however, and would likely be preferable in adults. These medications are indicated for treatment of hypertension, but have been noted to improve attention and decrease hyperactivity in children and adolescents with ADHD. These medications are typically dosed 2 to 3 times per day, which also limits their utility, but an extended-release form of guanfacine has been developed for which approval is being sought from the FDA for its use in children and adolescents.

Modafinil is a medication with an indication for use in narcolepsy to increase wakefulness in those with excessive daytime sleepiness. Clinical trials have shown modafinil to be effective for ADHD in children and adolescents, and an application for approval of an indication in this population was presented to the FDA; however, approval was not granted due to concerns about a number of reported cases of skin rash reactions in a 1,000-patient trial and what was believed to be one case of Stevens-Johnson syndrome (a potentially lethal skin reaction).

38. How does my doctor choose a class of medication to treat my ADHD?

As ADHD is a neurobiological disorder, the primary treatment modality of choice is pharmacological. Due to the high efficacy rate and generally good tolerability, the medication of choice is usually a stimulant, unless contraindicated, or if other factors make a given non-stimulant more desirable. Not only are stimulant medications very helpful for addressing the core ADHD symptoms, they work immediately once the effective dose level is reached. This is in contrast to many other medications used in the treatment of ADHD, which can take a month or more to demonstrate positive effects, not unlike the use of antidepressants in the treatment of major depression. Also, if one type of stimulant is tried and does not work, there is still a good chance that a stimulant of another formulation or type will be effective. If stimulants are not tolerated or are not helpful, then typically the next step is to try another type of medication, usually the non-stimulant, atomoxetine. Benefits of atomoxetine are described in Question 41. Other medications are utilized when stimulants and atomoxetine have not worked or when there are contraindications to their use, as well as when a comorbid condition necessitates the use of an alternative medication.

> *Not only are stimulant medications very helpful for addressing the core ADHD symptoms, they work immediately once the effective dose level is reached.*

39. How does my doctor choose a stimulant?

There are many choices of stimulants now available on the market, so it is reasonable to wonder how your doctor chooses one. For decades few choices were available, which limited their utility for many people. The stimulant dextroamphetamine was first used in the treatment of attention disorders in the 1930s and thus is one of the oldest medications in use for ADHD. Methylphenidate was developed in the 1960s and it, too, was widely used to treat ADHD in children. A characteristic of both stimulants, which were the only available treatments for ADHD for many years, was their short **half-life**, which meant that the body cleared them very quickly. Those medications, therefore, required dosing 2 to 3 times per day. Somewhat longer acting versions of both medications were eventually developed, but were found by many clinicians to be less effective than the short-acting medications. In 1996, however, a mixed amphetamine salt was introduced that, while also a short acting agent, exhibited less of the abrupt onset and termination of action than the single entity dextroamphetamine and lasted a couple hours longer per day. Then, in 2000, OROS-methylphenidate, a specially-designed controlled-release form of methylphenidate that lasted up to 12 hours, was developed, essentially revolutionizing the treatment of ADHD. No longer was midday dosing needed, and the gradual release and tapering of the stimulant was better tolerated. The introduction of OROS-methylphenidate into the market was closely followed by release of the mixed amphetamine salt extended-release capsule, so both classes of stimulants had an available option of an all-day coverage treatment. Since then, several other long-acting methylphenidate stimulants have been developed as well as an additional long-acting amphetamine agent. **Table 4** lists all the stimulants currently available and notes which ones are FDA approved for use in adult ADHD. The main differences among the medications have to do with the duration of action of the medication, the delivery system, and the distribution over the course of the day. The most recent addition to the stimulants is lisdexamfetamine, a pro-drug of dextroamphetamine. A pro-drug is inactive until it is digested in the gastrointestinal tract. The benefit of lisdexamfetamine is that there is less abuse potential due to the need for digestion of the drug in order for its active compound to be released.

Half-life

The time it takes for half of the blood concentration of a medication to be eliminated from the body. Half-life also determines the time to equilibrium of a drug in the blood and the frequency of dosing to achieve that equilibrium.

Table 4 Stimulants Available for Treatment of ADHD

Generic Name	Trade Name	Duration of Action**
Methylphenidate	Ritalin	3 to 4 hours
Methylphenidate ER	Ritalin SR	6 to 8 hours
Methylphenidate ER	Ritalin LA	8 hours
Methylphenidate ER	Metadate ER	6 to 8 hours
Methylphenidate ER	Metadate CD	8 hours
Methylphenidate ER	Concerta*	10 to 12 hours
D-Methylphenidate	Focalin	3 to 4 hours
D-Methylphenidate XR	Focalin XR*	12 to 14 hours
Methylphenidate TD (patch)	Daytrana	up to 12 hours
Dextroamphetamine	Dexedrine	4 to 5 hours
Dextroamphetamine ER	Dexedrine spansule	8 to 10 hours
Mixed amphetamine salts	Adderall	4 to 6 hours
Mixed amphetamine salts XR	Adderall XR*	10 to 12 hours
Lisdexamfetamine	Vyvanse*	12 to 14 hours

* These stimulant medications are FDA-approved for use in adults.
** Duration of Action is the average duration of active medication effect; this time period can vary between individuals.

In choosing a stimulant, a decision is made as to whether or not a long-acting agent should be prescribed. This is typical practice unless there are specific reasons to prescribe the short-acting medication. Because all stimulants are equally effective and have the same side effect profiles, the choice of stimulant is often based upon your physician's comfort with a particular agent. There are, however, good reasons to choose one over another, mainly due to duration of action and delivery system as noted in Table 4. Keep in mind that the medication's duration of action can vary from person to person based upon individual metabolism of the medication in question. Some individual considerations might include a need for more coverage hours or propensity for insomnia. For example, a 12-hour duration medication can provide needed coverage into the evening hours, but may be more likely to cause or exacerbate sleeplessness in some people than an 8-hour duration medication.

Short-acting stimulants can be tried if a long-acting formulation is not effective. The short-acting forms do have a sharper rise in blood levels, and some people may benefit more from that action, even though more frequent dosing is required. Mostly, however, short-acting agents are now utilized to cover the tail end of the day when the long-acting agent is wearing off. This is particularly important for people who work late hours or attend school in the evening. In contrast to the long-acting agents, short-acting agents are now available in generic forms, which may be preferable for some individuals from a financial standpoint.

Samantha comments,

When medications were first prescribed to me, it was basically trial and error. The medication targeted specific behaviors. Those were routinely assessed as to whether the medication was effective or not. I had tried several medications, both stimulants and nonstimulants. My body metabolizes medication quickly so it was necessary to make several increases of dosage when the most effective drug was determined. On an ongoing basis, my subjective experiences are continually evaluated.

Liza comments,

We have made changes based on my academic performance, mood, sleeping patterns, and daily functioning. I responded to the first stimulant my doctor prescribed and had few side effects. I maintain my weight, my vital signs are monitored, and I have been stable. My doctor has increased the dosage a few times and added a short-acting stimulant for when I need coverage later in the day.

40. How do the medications for ADHD work in the brain?

Either direct or indirect attenuation of dopamine and norepinephrine neurotransmission appears related to both the stimulant and nonstimulant medications efficacious in ADHD. However, important differences between the compounds exist. The stimulants methylphenidate and amphetamine are mostly similar in their mechanisms of action, both working by effectively increasing catecholamine circulation in the brain. Methylphenidate and amphetamine are norepinephrine and dopamine reuptake inhibitors, meaning they block the reuptake of norepinephrine and dopamine into the presynaptic neuron, thereby increasing circulating catecholamines in the synapse. Both compounds also increase the release of norepinephrine and dopamine from presynaptic vesicles into the synaptic cleft. Amphetamine has the additional action of directly stimulating postsynaptic dopaminergic receptors, which may account for its purported higher abuse liability.

Atomoxetine is a norepinephrine reuptake inhibitor only. It is this less direct action in the brain that likely accounts for the time frame needed before noticeable benefit is experienced with this medication. By changing the balance of norepinephrine in the brain, dopamine balance is adjusted because the two systems work in concert on the various frontal lobe functions. The tricyclic antidepressants and venlafaxine are thought to work in the same manner. Bupropion is thought to exert its effects via inhibition of dopamine reuptake. The anti-hypertensive medications, clonidine and guanfacine, exert their effects in the brain via their effects as alpha-2 **agonists,** which means that they directly stimulate the alpha-2 receptors located on the presynaptic neuron. These receptors help regulate the release of catecholamines from presynaptic vesicles. Studies in animals have shown that alpha-2 agonists improve cognitive abilities that arise from the prefrontal cortex. Modafinil's mechanism of action is uncertain but it

Agonist

A drug that binds to the receptor of a cell and triggers a response by the cell.

produces alterations in mood, perception, thinking, and feelings that are typical of other CNS stimulants.

41. How can I tell if the medication is working?

With stimulant medication it is usually quite clear when the medication starts to work, once an adequate dose is reached. Stimulants work for a specific time period, so their effects are often noticed to wear off at day's end as well. When taking a stimulant, the effects are rather robust and thus it is typically obvious to the person taking it that it is having a positive effect. Thinking often becomes clearer and more focused. Boredom may lift and energy levels increase. At the same time, it becomes easier to sit still. Self-rating scales can be useful to monitor for effects of medication as dosage adjustments are made as well.

With non-stimulants, you need to give these medications more time to exert their effects, and you need to be sure they are adequately dosed. Atomoxetine, for example, is dosed based upon weight. While the response to these medications does not appear as dramatic as when you take a stimulant each day, over time you can reassess your symptoms based upon your initial presentation to gauge improvement. Again, use of self-rating scales to monitor improvement can be very helpful, as it can be easy to forget the severity of some of the initial difficulties prior to starting treatment.

Samantha comments,

It is very obvious to me and others when I don't take my medication. My symptoms are immediately managed effectively when I take my medicine. Medication helps slow down my mind and body. I can listen and pay attention to myself and others. My thoughts slow down; my ability to sit, listen, and organize myself increases. I can prioritize better and can finish what I am doing. I become more social and at ease with myself. Ordinarily I struggle with writing things down, following directions of any kind, and shutting my mouth. A talker, I sometimes simply talk incessantly, repeating myself again and again, and don't allow others an opportunity to speak and respond to what I am saying. It can be difficult to communicate with me, and I can be exhausting to be around. As such, my friends and family also know when I didn't take my medication!

Liza comments,

When medication is working, my attention and concentration improves, my schoolwork assignments are managed, and I am able to study for greater lengths of time. When my medication wears off (early evening), it is difficult to maintain focus. When I need to prepare for a test or complete assignments, I take a short acting stimulant. Without that extra dose it is very difficult to prepare for a test, write papers, or tackle complex mathematics. Essentially, I can actually feel the medication kicking in. When I forget to take my medication I am easily frustrated and argumentative. My reactions are so much more intense when I am off medications. I cry easily and have zero patience for people, especially my family members. Life is more stressful in all areas, and I respond to situations with aggressiveness and anger. I am especially sensitive to criticism and become defensive for things that most people would not. Certainly, if I hadn't taken my medication I wouldn't be able to sit here and write the answers to these questions.

42. What are the benefits of atomoxetine?

Atomoxetine is the only nonstimulant medication approved for the treatment of ADHD in adults. Atomoxetine is a norepinephrine reuptake inhibitor, which means that the neurotransmitter norepinephrine is not taken back up into the presynaptic neuron, allowing for increasing circulating levels in the synaptic cleft. Atomoxetine has been shown in studies to reduce the symptoms of ADHD in contrast to **placebo**. Atomoxetine does, however, take 4 to 6 weeks to achieve full efficacy, which is why a stimulant is often the initial treatment of choice. In addition, atomoxetine needs to be taken every day to maintain adequate blood levels, in contrast to a stimulant,

Placebo

An inert substance that, when ingested, causes absolutely no physiological process to occur but may have psychological effects.

Atomoxetine takes 4 to 6 weeks to achieve full efficacy.

which can be stopped and restarted without affecting blood levels. The **effect size** of atomoxetine in studies is also not as high as that for stimulants, with a response rate of about 65% for atomoxetine. There are important benefits for atomoxetine however, so it is an important addition to treatment options available for ADHD. These benefits include:

Effect size

In research, indices that measure the magnitude of a treatment response.

- Coverage for 24 hours per day
- Less appetite reduction
- No abuse potential
- No exacerbation of underlying tic disorder
- Little to no exacerbation of underlying anxiety disorder
- Not a controlled substance and thus easier to obtain refills
- No rebound effects
- Possible dual coverage in the presence of a mood or anxiety disorder

Atomoxetine is also a good alternative for individuals who are unable to tolerate some of the side effects of stimulants or for whom they are simply ineffective. In certain situations, atomoxetine is indicated over a stimulant, such as in the presence of significant anxiety, when more constant coverage is desired or needed, if tics are present, or in the presence of substance abuse. If a stimulant is tried initially and is not helpful or not tolerable, then a trial of atomoxetine is warranted. Atomoxetine does have a warning on its labeling regarding its use in the presence of preexisting structural cardiac abnormalities or other serious heart problems, because sudden death has been associated with its use in children and adolescents who had such cardiac problems. There have been cases of stroke, myocardial infarction, and sudden death in adults who were on atomoxetine, but the role of atomoxetine in those cases is unknown.

43. How do I choose a therapist and a therapy approach?

Choosing a therapist can be an overwhelming task. One look in the yellow pages shows lists of names, and not everyone lists in the yellow pages. One factor to consider is the many possible credentials therapists can hold. Some people identify themselves as therapists but do not have credentials that require licensure within their states. In general, a licensed practitioner will have been through a screening process that usually involves testing within their field. Level of training is another consideration in choosing a therapist. There are master's levels (social workers), doctorate levels (psychologists), as well as medical doctorate levels (psychiatrists) who perform psychotherapy. Clinicians of various credentials may then have further training within a specific area of psychotherapy, such as psychoanalysis.

If you intend to take medication for ADHD and be in therapy, it may be useful to see a psychiatrist who also performs psychotherapy. Due to cost considerations, however, this option is not always feasible. Many insurance plans will provide reimbursement for a master's level therapist only and fees usually are less than those for psychologists or psychiatrists. If you have a specific treatment modality in mind, one method of finding a therapist is to obtain referrals from professional societies for that specific modality. If modality is not the issue of concern, referrals can be obtained from your primary care physician. You can speak with the therapist over the phone regarding initial questions and arrange a consultation. If you are uncomfortable with the therapist following the consultation, it is important to consider the reasons for your discomfort. Sometimes individual psychological issues are **projected** onto the therapist immediately and thus are avoided by failing to continue to see the therapist. But certainly you need to feel a fit with the therapist's style in order to develop a working relationship.

> *If you intend to take medication for ADHD and be in therapy, it may be useful to see a psychiatrist who also performs psychotherapy.*

Projection

The attribution of one's own unconscious thoughts and feelings to others.

44. What are the different talk therapies and how do they work for ADHD?

Once you receive a consultation, the clinician will make recommendations as to the most appropriate treatment or therapeutic approach for your circumstances. He or she may be able to utilize that approach or refer you to persons who specialize in that specific approach. Many therapists utilize a combination of therapeutic approaches in their work. Some of the different approaches are outlined here.

Psychodynamic therapy assumes presenting symptoms are due to unresolved, **unconscious** conflicts from childhood. It is based upon the classic psychoanalytic approach developed by Sigmund Freud. The therapist uses the concepts of **transference**, **countertransference**, **resistance**, free association, and dreams in order to help the patient develop insight into patterns in relationships that can then effect change. It is a nondirective therapy. While classic analytical therapy can last for years, with sessions four to five days per week, psychodynamic therapy may be shorter in duration, with sessions one to three times per week. Controlled research studies examining the efficacy of this type of therapy are minimal, due to the nature of this type of therapy. It is often a helpful treatment approach for those with chronic coping difficulties or with **personality disorders** and would not necessarily be considered a treatment to address ADHD symptoms specifically.

Interpersonal therapy (IPT) was developed as a treatment approach for depression, conceptualizing depression in a patient with the three components of symptom formation, social functioning, and personality factors. Interpersonal therapy focuses on the patient's social, or interpersonal, functioning, with expected improvement in symptoms. The goal is to improve communication skills and self-esteem. It is a brief and highly structured, manual-based psychotherapy. Areas of social functioning that may be addressed are interpersonal disputes, role transitions, grief, and interpersonal deficits. Therapy is focused and brief in duration, typically lasting 12 to 16 sessions. Research studies have shown it to be an effective treatment for depression.

Cognitive behavioral therapy (CBT) is utilized in a variety of mood and anxiety disorders. The theory presumes symptoms can occur as a result of a pattern of negative thinking. It works

Psychodynamic

Referring to a type of therapy that focuses on one's interpersonal relationships, developmental experiences, and the transference relationship with his or her therapist.

Unconscious

An underlying motivation for behavior that has developed over the course of life experience and is not available to the conscious or thoughtful mind.

Transference

The unconscious assignment of feelings and attitudes to a therapist from previous important relationships in one's life (parents and siblings).

Countertransference

The attitudes, opinions, and behaviors that a therapist attributes to his or her patient, not based on the true nature of the patient but rather the biased nature of the therapist because the patient reminds the therapist of his or her own past relationships.

to help patients identify and change inaccurate perceptions of themselves and situations. It also is brief in duration and manual-based, typically lasting for 10 to 20 sessions. It typically involves the use of homework assignments between sessions. Research studies have shown it to be an effective treatment for depression and anxiety disorders, and while there is no evidence for its use as a replacement for pharmacotherapy, it is being adapted for use as an adjunctive treatment for ADHD. Question 44 describes cognitive behavioral therapy more in depth.

45. What is cognitive behavioral therapy and how can it be used for ADHD?

Cognitive behavioral therapy is based upon two separate theoretical models, both cognitive and behavioral. Cognitive models are based upon the premise that **cognitions**, or thoughts, determine emotions and behavior. **Automatic thoughts** are one type of cognition that may be distorted by errors of thinking such as **overgeneralization**, **catastrophic thinking**, jumping to conclusions, or personalization. Errors in thinking tend to be more frequent and intense in depression as well as in other psychiatric disorders. Behavioral models are based upon theories of learning such as by **modeling** or by reinforcement to certain responses.

Cognitive behavioral therapy is an approach that uses techniques based upon the models described above. A greater emphasis on cognitive approaches or on behavioral approaches may be taken depending upon the disorder and the stage of treatment. Cognitive techniques include:

- Psychoeducation
- Modifying automatic thoughts
- Modifying **schemas**

Behavioral techniques include:

- Activity scheduling
- Breathing control

Treatment

Resistance

The tendency to avoid treatment interventions, often unconsciously (e.g., missed appointments, arriving late, forgetting medication).

Personality disorder

Maladaptive behavior patterns that persist throughout the life span causing functional impairments.

Interpersonal therapy

A form of therapy. Unlike psychodynamic therapy that focuses on developmental relationships, interpersonal therapy focuses strictly on current relationships and conflicts within them.

Cognitive behavioral therapy

A combination of cognitive and behavioral approaches in psychotherapy, during which the therapist focuses on automatic thoughts and behavior of a self-defeating quality in order to make one more conscious of them and replace them with more positive thoughts and behaviors.

Cognitions

The mental processes of knowing, thinking, learning, and judging.

Automatic thoughts

Thoughts that occur spontaneously whenever a specific, common event occurs in one's life, and that are often associated with depression.

Overgeneralization

The act of taking a specific event, usually one that was psychologically traumatic, and applying one's reactions to that event to an ever-increasing array of events that are not really in the same class but are perceived as such.

Catastrophic thinking

A type of automatic thought during which the individual quickly assumes the worst outcome for a given situation.

Modeling

Learning that occurs from observation.

- **Contingency contracting**
- Desensitization/relaxation training
- Exposure and **flooding**
- Social skills training
- Thought stopping/distraction

Through many of these techniques, patients learn to appropriately manage anxiety and reactions to stress. Exposure training is a technique that uses **graded exposure** to a high-anxiety situation by breaking the task into small steps that are focused on one by one.

CBT has been the best-studied form of psychotherapy, and has been shown to effectively treat depression and many anxiety disorders. Safren et al. (2004) developed a cognitive behavioral treatment for adults receiving pharmacological treatment of ADHD who continue to have residual, impairing symptoms. The modules that were developed addressed:

- Organization and planning
- Coping with distractibility
- Cognitive restructuring
- Procrastination
- Anger management
- Communication skills

While there is no evidence that CBT can be used to treat ADHD symptoms in the absence of medication, it can be used to treat residual symptoms. CBT treatment typically lasts three to six months with 10 to 20 weekly sessions. The patient is expected to be an active participant in trying out new strategies and is typically expected to do homework. CBT techniques can also focus on changing cognitions, goal setting, and development of compensatory strategies.

46. What is coaching and how can it help with ADHD?

Coaching is a method of directing, instructing, and training a person or group of people, with the aim of achieving some goal or developing specific skills. The practice of coaching is non-directive, serving to help clients analyze and solve their own challenges, rather than offer advice or direction. Life coaches help clients determine and achieve personal goals. Coaching is not targeted at psychological illness and coaches are not therapists.

ADD coaches specialize in working with clients with ADHD, supporting them in developing a comprehensive understanding of both the nature of ADHD and its impact on quality of life. ADD coaches create structure, support, skills, and strategies to help clients develop more satisfying lives. Coaching can help clients address core ADHD-related issues like time management, organization, and self-esteem. The ADD coach can help clients:

- Develop an increased understanding of the neurobiological nature of ADHD
- Understand the source of many of their challenges is not due to personal shortcomings
- Examine areas of failure and areas where they want to be held accountable
- Reframe the ADHD, creating a new awareness that explains past underperformance, thereby diminishing self-blame
- Heighten self-awareness and self-observation skills, and use those heightened skills to improve decision-making and performance
- Change perspective when "stuck" (e.g., learning new ways to work with procrastination, perfectionism, and staying on task, and learning to be more consistent)
- Become aware of their own learning styles, processing styles, and learning preferences

Treatment

Schema

The internal representation of the world that each person holds, which can be revised as new information is obtained.

Contingency contracting

A behavioral therapy technique that utilizes reinforcers or rewards to modify behavior.

Flooding

A behavioral therapy technique that involves exposure to the maximal level of anxiety as quickly as possible.

Graded exposure

A psychotherapeutic technique applied to rid a patient of specific phobias. A gradual exposure to the phobic situation is set about first through imagery techniques and then with limited exposure in time and intensity before full exposure occurs.

Coaching

A practice of helping clients determine and achieve personal goals.

Coaching is not a therapy, but can be an adjunctive treatment to an existing therapy or can be used alone if therapy is not considered indicated.

While coaching is not a therapy, it can be an adjunctive treatment to an existing therapy or can be used alone if therapy is not indicated. Although it has become an increasingly recognized method of helping adults with ADHD, keep in mind that since it is not a therapy, it is not covered by insurance. Licensure for coaching varies in different states, so it is important to check on credentials and experience of a coach. Some coaches have clinical backgrounds such as in social work or psychology, but have changed careers or are working in both capacities in their practice.

47. How can psychotherapy work if ADHD is due to a chemical imbalance?

Remission

Complete cessation of all symptoms associated with a specific mental illness, which can be temporary or permanent.

While psychotherapy can facilitate the attainment of **remission** for some psychiatric disorders, such as depression, when it comes to ADHD, the symptoms of ADHD do not "go into remission" with therapy. Some forms of psychotherapy, such as CBT or IPT, have even been found to be as good as medication for the treatment of mild to moderate major depression and CBT is used successfully for many anxiety disorders, such as generalized anxiety or obsessive-compulsive disorder. While depression and anxiety disorders have associated heritability, there is a greater degree of environmental influence on the development and persistence of those disorders than there is for ADHD. To date, there is no evidence of psychotherapy being as good as medication for the core symptoms of ADHD. However, many of the functional impairments that occur secondary to core ADHD symptoms can be responsive to therapy because the development of coping strategies can reduce those impairments. Psychotherapy facilitates the same changes in the brain that are seen to occur in response to learning, so therapy can help correct some of the functional responses to ADHD that have become maladaptive. For example, low frustration tolerance is common in ADHD, consistent with symptoms of impulsivity. The loss of temper that often occurs with that frustration can be addressed as a maladaptive coping style in psychotherapy.

Psychotherapy in ADHD patients can address the sequelae of the core ADHD symptoms, such as failed performance in work or school and failed relationships. Living with ADHD can result in chronic low self-esteem. Many adults have grown up with the belief that they were lazy, unmotivated, and stupid. These issues can be successfully addressed through psychotherapy. In addition, ADHD is often associated with other disorders with rates of major depression and **dysthymic disorder** higher than in the general population, as well as anxiety disorders, bipolar disorder, and substance abuse. All these comorbid conditions benefit from psychotherapy.

48. What is behavioral modification?

Behavioral modification is a treatment intervention commonly used in children and adolescents that essentially rewards desired behavior with privileges or rewards and discourages unwanted behavior with removal of privileges or adding consequences. A typical structure for children is to use a reward chart with use of stickers or stars indicating achieved goals. For adolescents, points may be given that can be redeemed for items or time for enjoyed activities (television, computer). Behavioral modification techniques have been demonstrated in research studies to be beneficial both alone and as an adjunctive treatment to medication for ADHD (thus resulting in a more robust response). At face value, it would not appear that behavioral modification could be of use in the adult population; however, individuals can utilize the premise of behavioral modification in implementing a program. Behavioral techniques used in adults might include the use of tools such as personal digital assistants, schedulers, and to-do lists; organization of the home to include specific areas for keys, wallet, etc.; forming of strategies to reduce jumping into activities without thinking; and planning what to say for anticipated situations. Create goals for yourself that are achievable, such as spending 30 minutes on a given task. When you complete a goal, reward yourself with an enjoyable activity or item.

Dysthymic disorder

A type of depressive disorder that is characterized by the presence of chronic, mild depressive symptoms.

Treatment

49. What are the side effects of medications used to treat ADHD?

Side effects occur with all medications, not just psychotropic medications. In the treatment of ADHD, however, medications are taken for long periods, so some side effects may not be tolerable due to the duration of treatment required. Side effects vary both within a class of medications and between classes. Typically, one class of medications shares similar side effects; however, if one medicine within a class causes a specific side effect (e.g., nausea), it is not necessarily the case that another medicine within the same class will cause the same side effect.

Table 5 lists some of the more common side effects from specific medication classes. Some medications have rare, but serious, side effects that have been reported. Your doctor should go over any of these with you. In the case of stimulants, while the safety profile is generally good, there can be heightened risk for cardiac complications in the presence of underlying cardiac disease (Question 48) or if taken concomitantly with illicit substances.

Rather than discontinuing a medication when there is a suspected bothersome side effect, it is important to speak with your doctor first. Some side effects are transient or can be easily alleviated by another remedy (e.g., ibuprofen for headache) and some side effects can be managed by changing the dosing schedule or by changing to a medication with a shorter duration of action, such as when insomnia occurs. With some types of medication, stopping them abruptly when any side effect occurs may cause a **discontinuation syndrome**, or may prematurely interrupt a potentially helpful treatment intervention. If possible, it is best to remain on a treatment for at least a few days because some perceived side effects could be associated with unrelated conditions (e.g., tension headache). Bear in mind, scientific studies that compare an active medication to a placebo (sugar pill) have reported "side effects" in

Discontinuation syndrome

Physical symptoms that occur when a drug is suddenly stopped.

Table 5   Adverse Effects of Medication used in the Treatment of ADHD*

Medication (listed *by group* or individually)	Potential Adverse Effects
Stimulants	reduced appetite, nausea, insomnia, nervousness, agitation, abdominal pain, dry mouth, headache, dizziness, tachycardia, elevated blood pressure, irritability
Atomoxetine	dry mouth, reduced appetite, dizziness, fatigue, insomnia, constipation, nausea, headache, depression, irritability, decreased libido, erectile difficulty, hepatic failure (rare)
Bupropion	weight loss, dry mouth, rash, sweating, agitation, dizziness, insomnia, nausea, abdominal pain, weakness, headache, blurred vision, constipation, tremor, rapid heart rate, ringing in ears, seizures
Venlafaxine	sweating, nausea, constipation, decreased appetite, vomiting, insomnia, somnolence, dry mouth, dizziness, nervousness, tremor, blurred vision, sexual dysfunction, rapid heart rate, hypertension
Tricyclic antidepressants	dry mouth, constipation, nausea, anorexia, weight gain, sweating, increased appetite, nervousness, decreased libido, dizziness, tremor, somnolence, blurred vision, tachycardia, urinary hesitancy, hypotension, cardiac toxicity
Anti-hypertensives	dizziness, drowsiness, constipation, depression, headache, nausea, vomiting, dry mouth
Modafinil	headache, infection, nausea, nervousness, anxiety, insomnia

* Listed adverse effects are not exhaustive of side effects as reported in the *Physicians' Desk Reference*. Rather more common effects within each group were included, as well as some more serious effects. Side effect profiles of medications within a class may vary. Any concern about an adverse effect from a medication should be discussed with your doctor.

the placebo group as well. That said, if a suspected effect seems dangerous for any reason, it is certainly most prudent to stop the medication until you are able to speak with your doctor and, if necessary, get evaluated in an emergency setting.

50. What are the cardiac risks associated with stimulants?

Stimulants are known to have modest effects on the cardiovascular system, namely increasing the blood pressure and heart rate. These effects are typically mild, however, and any

Stimulants are known to have modest effects on the cardiovascular system, namely increasing the blood pressure and heart rate.

increase that occurs is not significant for most people (heart rate increased by 1 to 2 beats per minute and blood pressure by 3 to 4 mm Hg). From 1999 to 2003, 19 sudden deaths and 26 cardiovascular events were reported in children and adolescents who were taking stimulant medications. The rate of these events was no different than in the general population. With that data in mind, however, the FDA changed the labeling on all stimulants to indicate a risk of cardiovascular complications including sudden death in individuals with preexisting structural cardiac abnormalities or other serious heart problems. The standard practice has been to evaluate for cardiac disease by review of symptoms and history. If an individual had symptoms suggestive of a cardiac abnormality or a family history for sudden cardiac death, further work-up has been recommended prior to initiation of a stimulant. More recently, however, the American Heart Association conducted a review and analysis of these cardiovascular risks to determine the utility of screening **electrocardiograms** in children and adolescents prior to starting stimulants. Since the most common cardiac abnormalities in children and adolescents that can lead to sudden death can be detected via electrocardiogram (ECG), it has been recommended that screening ECGs for children and adolescents who are to start or who have been taking stimulants be considered. As the tests are non-invasive with little risk (the risk of screening ECGs is getting a false positive, which can result in unnecessary anxiety and expense in getting a full cardiac workup), the benefit of identifying any asymptomatic cardiac disease is emphasized. The recommendation, however, remains mired in controversy within the medical community due to the level of evidence used in making the recommendation.

While the recommendation by the American Heart Association was not geared toward the adult population specifically, it makes sense to consider screening ECGs in this population for the same reasons, especially since cardiovascular disease risk rises with age through adulthood. An abnormal ECG does not rule out the use of a stimulant, however. A cardiologist

Electrocardiogram

A noninvasive recording of the electrical activity of the heart.

will typically be consulted for guidance and, based upon the clinical impression, there may not be a contraindication to taking a stimulant.

51. Are there long-term dangers to taking medication?

Around for decades, stimulants have a long track record of safety with long-term use with no evidence for any long-term dangers related to stimulants. One longstanding concern has been the stimulants' effects on growth of children because recent studies have shown evidence for a lag in height growth relative to control subjects, the rate of which appears to decrease over time. Growth concerns would not be an issue for adults, however. Another issue that has arisen as a potential long-term risk would be whether use of stimulants could predispose the patient to abuse of alcohol or drugs. This concern has not been founded in studies, however (see Question 50). The main risk of concern in the adult population is the cardiovascular effects that result from stimulants, which are discussed in Question 48. While there are no other documented long-term adverse effects from stimulants, your doctor may want to monitor functioning of some organ systems with periodic blood work. People with certain conditions, such as hyperthyroidism, glaucoma, and moderate to severe hypertension, should not take stimulants because these conditions can be worsened.

Labeling was added to atomoxetine following post-marketing reports of two cases of liver injury that resulted from atomoxetine. The two cases were out of an estimated 2 million prescriptions for atomoxetine, so this potential adverse effect is considered rare. Both of the patients with liver injury recovered after atomoxetine was discontinued. It is recommended that immediate evaluation be undertaken if symptoms of liver injury such as **jaundice**, nausea and vomiting, right-sided upper abdominal pain, flulike symptoms, or dark urine occur. In addition, atomoxetine has labeling of potential cardiovascular

Jaundice

Yellow staining of the skin and sclerae of the eyes due to abnormally high levels of bilirubin, which typically indicates liver or gallbladder disease.

risk similar to stimulants (as discussed in Question 48) in persons with preexisting structural cardiac abnormalities or other heart problems. Stroke, sudden death, and heart attacks have occurred in adults who are taking atomoxetine; however, the role of atomoxetine in those cases is not known.

Atomoxetine also has an FDA warning for increased risk for suicidal ideation in children and adolescents. This risk is low as well, but you should be aware of it and inform your doctor right away if you start experiencing suicidal thoughts. All antidepressants have this labeling regarding suicide risk, including increased risk in young adults, so the same risk would apply to antidepressants being used for ADHD, although studies that document the small increase in suicidal ideation are studies done primarily on depressed patients.

52. Can I become addicted to the medication?

The one major concern for many patients who take medications for years is the fear that they can become addicted to the medication. **Addiction** is a complicated and controversial issue that bears some explaining. From a medical standpoint, addiction is defined as pursuit of a substance in such a manner that the pursuit and use of it consumes so much time and energy for the person to the exclusion of the majority of, if not all of, the important activities in that person's life.

The stimulants are a controlled substance, meaning they have been identified as a class of medication having potential for abuse. When a medication is presented to the FDA for approval, a determination is made as to whether the drug in question needs to be controlled. The Comprehensive Drug Abuse Prevention and Control Act of 1970 established the mechanism of determining placement of a medication under the jurisdiction of the DEA, utilizing criteria such as the medication's actual or relative potential for abuse, the scientific evidence of its pharmacological effect, the medication's history and current pattern of abuse, and its **dependence** liability.

Addiction

Continued use of a mood-altering substance despite physical, psychological, or social harm. It is characterized by a lack of control in the amount and frequency of use, cravings, continued use in the presence of adverse effects, denial of negative consequences, and a tendency to abuse other mood-altering substances.

The one major concern for many patients who take medications for years is the fear that they can become addicted to the medication.

Dependence

The body's reliance on a drug to function normally. Physical dependence results in withdrawal when the drug is stopped suddenly. Dependence should be contrasted to addiction.

Once determined that a medication should be controlled, it is placed into one of five schedules on the basis of its potential for abuse, accepted medical use, and accepted safety under medical supervision. Substances listed as Schedule I have a high potential for abuse, no accredited medical use, and a lack of accepted safety. From Schedules I to V, substances decrease in potential for abuse, with methylphenidate and amphetamine compounds listed as Schedule II controlled substances.

Although considered to have abuse potential, stimulants are not in and of themselves addicting if used as prescribed—that is, you will be able to discontinue the medication without difficulty if it is being taken as prescribed. If taken in excessive amounts for other purposes, such as to get high or to stay awake, then there is increasing potential for addiction, that is, to continue to seek the drug for its mood-elevating effects. In addition, use of the medication via methods other than oral ingestion (e.g., inhalation) will create heightened risk for addiction. Due to these risks, the use of stimulants is not recommended for individuals who have active substance abuse. It is somewhat controversial whether or not stimulants can be prescribed to those with histories of substance abuse who are currently in remission. It may be more prudent to try a non-controlled medication first, but bear in mind that untreated ADHD is a risk factor for abuse of drugs, and thus when treated appropriately and under a doctor's supervision, the risk for substance abuse may markedly decrease. Similar worries people have for heightened risk of substance abuse in general are unfounded, as recent studies have not found elevated risks for adult substance abuse in children who were treated with stimulants. There continues to be speculation that treatment may actually lower the risk for substance abuse; however, this specific finding has not been documented in studies thus far. As the presence of ADHD is a known risk for later substance abuse, more studies are needed to look at the impact treatment has on these risks.

Treatment

The recently developed stimulant pro-drug, lisdexamfetamine, is thought to have lower abuse potential due to the necessity for gastrointestinal digestion to release its active compound. It has been found to have low "likability," one factor taken into account when a drug is evaluated for its abuse potential; however, it remains a Schedule II drug at this time, as are other stimulants.

53. I feel irritable and lethargic when my medication wears off at the end of the day. What can I do about it?

As the stimulant medication wears off at the end of the day, a phenomenon known as stimulant rebound can occur. This was more common when short-acting stimulants were primarily in use, and often manifested in children as deterioration in behavior. Irritability, tearfulness, and higher-than-baseline hyperactivity are typical features of stimulant rebound. In adults, irritability and lethargy may occur as the stimulant wears off, along with recurrence of ADHD symptoms, which can be difficult to readjust to. The long-acting preparations of stimulants are less likely to result in rebound effects, but these effects can still occur. One solution is to add a short-acting stimulant at a lesser dosage at the end of the day to continue covering the ADHD symptoms and lessen the experience of lethargy and irritability. Other options would be to try another formulation of your stimulant that has a different medication distribution across the day, or to try a different stimulant. If the wearing-off effects continue and are bothersome, 24-hour coverage with a non-stimulant medication might be preferable.

54. What can I do about weight loss from taking medication?

One of the more common side effects of stimulant medications used to treat ADHD is loss of appetite. As a consequence, weight loss can sometimes occur. The appetite loss is associated with the duration of action of the medication, so typically the peak appetite suppression is during the day. As

One of the more common side effects of stimulant medications used to treat ADHD is loss of appetite.

the medication wears off by evening, appetite usually returns. You can take advantage of the evening appetite rebound by increasing caloric intake at this time, having dinner later if necessary. Other strategies to manage loss of appetite include eating a full breakfast before the medication effects kick in and then eating small snacks during the day, even if not particularly hungry. After some time, the loss of appetite side effect will often wane.

Sometimes, significant weight loss can occur and strategies to take in food do not adequately offset this weight loss. In this case, a reduced medication dosage or change to a shorter duration of action of medication may be helpful. In certain circumstances, alternatives to a stimulant may be necessary. The loss of appetite that can occur with atomoxetine may not be as great and some of the other treatments do not commonly have loss of appetite as a side effect.

55. Are there any natural remedies for ADHD?

"Natural" or **alternative treatments** describe any treatment that has not been scientifically documented or identified as safe or effective for a certain medical condition. Examples of alternative treatments include acupuncture, yoga, herbal remedies, aromatherapy, biofeedback, and many others. In considering an alternative treatment, as with any scientifically documented treatment, one should consider the risks versus the benefits of such a treatment. If a particular procedure has no specific, direct risks associated with it, one important risk is potentially delayed treatment. Depending upon the circumstances for which you are coming in to be evaluated for symptoms secondary to ADHD, you may feel that it is imperative to have relief as soon as possible. This may be the case if there are significant work-related or intimate relationship difficulties. The medications indicated for ADHD have fairly rapid efficacy and it is possible that trials of untested treatments will result in further delay.

Alternative treatment

A treatment for a medical condition that has not undergone scientific studies to demonstrate its efficacy.

Other risks of alternative treatments include loss of money on an ineffective treatment, use of a treatment that is not standardized nor required to conform to specific regulations, and frustration when hopes of a unique treatment are not realized.

Herbal remedies are a popular "natural" choice for treatment of many conditions. A common assumption about these types of treatment choices is that they are safe because they are natural. While herbs are found in nature, as with manmade chemicals, herbs have a specific chemical structure that also alters the body chemistry. As such, there can be significant side effects from such compounds as well. Some of these side effects can be life threatening. For example, there have been many cases of liver failure from use of kava supplements around the world. In many cases, the problem is not that there are side effects per se, but that the herbal treatments are not regulated as to either their safety or efficacy. If a specific treatment is known to be effective, there may be certain risks one is willing to take for relief. But without known efficacy it is not possible to make an informed decision as to the risks from exposure. Lack of regulation also means supplements available in the store are not rigorously tested for purity or quantity of the active compound in question. Individuals who sell these treatments may act as experts, but have not necessarily obtained any specialized training or certification either. It is important to keep these issues in mind when undertaking an alternative treatment, so that you can make fully informed decisions about treatment. If you do decide to try an alternative treatment, it is important to communicate this information with your doctor. Herbal treatments in particular may interact with other medications, making it especially important to do so.

Supplements used to target ADHD symptoms include gingko biloba and omega fatty acids. There has been research on the use of omega fatty acids; however, to date the results of its efficacy for ADHD are not encouraging.

EEG biofeedback is considered an alternative treatment that has been found to have efficacy in some studies. It is discussed in more detail in Question 56.

56. What is EEG biofeedback and how is it used to treat ADHD?

Biofeedback is a type of treatment in which patients are taught to control physiological functions such as heart rate, muscle tension, and brain waves. Studies on its use for ADHD are sparse and many include only a small number of patients. It is thought that with biofeedback, ADHD patients can learn to increase activity in the regions of the brain involved in sustained attention, focus, and problem solving. In EEG biofeedback, ADHD patients will unconsciously decrease slow wave activity or increase fast wave activity in their brains. **Positive reinforcement** is utilized to achieve this goal. In a treatment session, electrodes are placed on the patient's head and connected to a computer. When a certain brain pattern is detected by the computer, a monitor being watched by the patient will respond, such as with points or with movement of game characters. The theory is that, over time, the brain will learn to produce the normal EEG patterns on its own and thus correct the abnormalities that cause ADHD symptoms. Some studies have shown improvement in academic performance in children, but it is not known how these improvements generalize to other settings or if improvements were due to other factors. EEG biofeedback requires 20 to 60 sessions, that typically occur over a time frame of a year, and can be costly. Insurance companies do not reimburse for the procedure. It is not known if any improvements in the course of these treatments are sustained beyond the treatment period.

Positive reinforcement

The presentation of something rewarding or pleasurable immediately following a behavior that makes it more likely the behavior will occur again.

57. Will diet or exercise help alleviate my ADHD symptoms?

There have been longstanding claims that artificially added flavors, coloring, and preservatives, as well as excessive sugar in food, can exacerbate ADHD. While there have been a few positive studies, mainly of young children showing increased activity or slightly reduced attention, scientifically controlled studies have not supported the theory that additives cause normal children to develop ADHD or that children with ADHD are worsened in their symptoms. Elimination diets have been found valid in only a small subset of patients with food allergies, and such food sensitivities are considered uncommon. As far as sugar is concerned, several studies done over the past couple of decades have mainly proven to be negative. While a healthy, well-rounded diet is a good idea for overall well-being, there is no evidence that following a particular diet plan can help with ADHD symptoms.

As for exercise, there are many theories as to how it improves mental health in general. Exercise causes changes in levels of serotonin, norepinephrine, and dopamine and causes the release of **endorphins** (which mask pain). Exercise may reduce muscle tension, and adrenaline is released, which counteracts effects of stress. Psychologically, too, exercise improves self-esteem, provides structure and routine, increases social contacts, and distracts from daily stress. Yoga is a type of exercise that also emphasizes self-awareness to promote a mind-body connection that may facilitate self-control. The relaxation techniques that are learned can be utilized when feeling out of control or overwhelmed. While the degree of impact that exercise has on ADHD needs more research, there are many good reasons for including regular exercise as part of a treatment plan for ADHD.

58. What is educational therapy?

Educational therapy is an intervention combining educational and therapeutic approaches for evaluation, remediation, case management, and advocacy on behalf of children, adolescents, and adults. The educational therapist works with clients who have learning disabilities or learning problems such as dyslexia, ADHD, language processing, or math problems as

Endorphins

Chemicals produced by the body that serve to suppress pain.

Educational therapy

An education intervention that investigates, defines, and addresses an individual's pattern of learning.

Yoga is a type of exercise that also emphasizes self-awareness to promote a mind-body connection that may facilitate self-control. The relaxation techniques that are learned can be utilized when feeling out of control or overwhelmed.

well as problems with academic self-esteem, motivation, organization, and study skills. Educational therapists may work with students who need appropriate school placements or adults needing school or workplace support. Services provided by educational therapists include:

- Formal and informal educational assessments
- Synthesis of information from other specialists
- Development and implementation of remedial programs for school-related learning and behavior problems
- Strategy training for addressing social and emotional aspects of learning problems
- Facilitation of communication between the individual, family, school, and involved professionals.

An educational therapist may be certified by the Association of Educational Therapists or from a four-year university program offering a certificate in the program. Many educational therapists have master's degrees or have completed the equivalent graduate level work. The Association of Educational Therapists offers board certification in educational therapy when certain criteria are met.

59. My medication is not helping. What happens next?

Steps to be taken when a given medication is not providing results depend upon what has already been tried. While stimulants are the most effective medication treatment for ADHD, they do not work for everyone. In studies, the response rate is between 70% and 80%, a very good rate but still not covering everyone. For non-responders to the first stimulant tried, trial of another stimulant outside the subclass results in increased rates of response, so a switch from a methylphenidate to an amphetamine compound or vice versa is usually indicated. Also, it is possible that a switch within a class can be helpful, due to the differing **pharmacokinetic**

Pharmacokinetic

The process by which a drug is absorbed, distributed, metabolized, and eliminated by the body.

Treatment

profiles of each formulation. Also important is that the dosage is maximized as high as tolerated. Frequently "nonresponse" can actually be attributed to inadequate dosing that is well below the maximum recommended dosage. Even with the FDA-recommended maximum dosage, however, many clinicians find that higher doses are indicated for some individuals and, under close monitoring, are able to bring their dose up to more effective levels. The FDA recommendation is typically based upon dosages used in studies, but once a medication is introduced into public use, there can be a higher variation of effective dosing range. If, however, stimulants are not found effective, the next medication of choice is usually atomoxetine. While the response rate tends to be lower (about 65%) than for stimulants, it can be effective for a stimulant non-responder because it works via a different mechanism. An adequate trial of atomoxetine is four to six weeks at a dosage based upon body weight (typical dosing is between 1.2 and 1.4 mg/kg).

If both stimulants and atomoxetine have been unsuccessful, other off-label choices can be considered as noted in Question 37. In addition, the diagnosis should be reassessed to check for previously missed comorbid conditions, as untreated depression, anxiety, or other conditions may make the response to ADHD treatments rather limited. In addition, be sure to be up front with your clinician regarding any substance use. It is not uncommon for people with ADHD to use substances such as marijuana to relax; however, its usage can render any treatments ineffective.

60. Will the medication turn me into a zombie or make me look drugged up?

Looking "medicated" is often a reason why some people avoid treatment with psychotropic medications. While some medications used in psychiatric practice can affect a person's state of alertness, perhaps making that person look robotic or overly sedated, stimulants do not cause this effect. Sometimes individuals can feel slowed down or lower in energy, usually because the hyperactivity and restlessness they normally experience is reduced. If too marked a feeling of slowing occurs, a reduction of the dosage of medication will likely be helpful. If not, then a switch to another agent can be tried. No one should be able to tell by your appearance that you are taking medication, although some may notice a difference in your behavior when symptoms are improved.

Some worry their personality will be changed by medication. Medication does not change a personality. Aside from the presence of side effects, you should experience no specific effects on personality from ADHD medications. Inasmuch as many adults have been living with ADHD without treatment for many, many years, it can feel as if their personality is being altered. Also, many persons can tell when the medication is kicking in and when it is wearing off, but this is not characterized by an appearance of being medicated.

Liza comments,

To the contrary, when I am not taking Adderall I can look "spacey." My mind wanders and I daydream a lot. To others it looks like I am not paying attention. I also stare at others without realizing it. I am not hyperactive.

61. My medication is helping, but I have side effects. What can I do?

If your medication is helpful but some side effects are bothersome, there may be some techniques to help alleviate the adverse effects. The most common side effect of stimulants is loss of appetite and subsequent weight loss. It is important to keep any weight loss in perspective, for as long as you remain in the appropriate weight range for your height, this is not usually a problem. The weight loss will usually stop at some point and then weight will remain stable. Ways around the appetite suppression include taking advantage of the times medication is not on board to consume calories. Have a big breakfast, expecting to have a light or no lunch, and then eat dinner when the medication has worn off, even if it is later

No one should be able to tell by your appearance that you are taking medication, although some may notice a difference in your behavior when symptoms are improved.

Treatment

than your typical evening meal. Also, try to eat small, healthy snacks, even when not hungry during the day, knowing that it is the medication that is suppressing your appetite. If your appetite does not return at the latter end of the evening, then you might want to consider a shorter acting stimulant that wears off earlier in the day. Also, for many people, the appetite suppression does dissipate with time, so patience for this may be all that is needed.

For insomnia, the best course is to consider a stimulant that is shorter in duration of action, or to try taking the medication earlier, such as immediately upon awakening in the morning. For stomach upset, the medicine can be taken with food. Sometimes a dosage can be reduced a small amount and still be effective, but not have side effects. Lastly, if the side effects remain problematic, it is useful to try another stimulant, either within the same class or of the other class. While side effect profiles are the same, the adverse effects can vary from person to person depending upon delivery system or type of stimulant.

62. Can I take other medications with ADHD medications?

When taking any medication, be sure to inform all your doctors of them. Some medications can cause adverse reactions as a result of their combination. Some lose their effectiveness in the presence of another medication or break down more slowly, necessitating a lower dosage. That said, not many medications have adverse interactions with stimulants. The one class of medications that is contraindicated with stimulants is the monoamine oxidase (MAO) inhibitors. These antidepressants are used much less commonly than years ago, and are considered only when other antidepressant treatments have failed. The combination of MAO inhibitors and psychostimulants can result in headaches, a **hypertensive crisis**, and **hyperpyrexia** as a result of the release of increased catecholamine stores. For the same reason, atomoxetine should not be taken with MAO inhibitors. Atomoxetine may require dosage

Hypertensive crisis

A condition characterized by extremely high blood pressure levels.

Hyperpyrexia

Abnormally high fever.

adjustments when prescribed with certain SSRIs, specifically those **metabolized** via a certain enzyme system in the liver, as the metabolism of atomoxetine is reduced which causes blood levels to go up and may also cause increased side effects. For venlafaxine, in addition to MAO inhibitors being contraindicated, caution should be used in combination with other agents that prolong the cardiac **QT interval**. Combination with other serotonergic agents, such as SSRI antidepressants or sibutramine, can result in the **serotonin syndrome**.

63. How do I know if I should see a specialist?

Many clinicians can diagnose and treat ADHD, including different physician specialists. That said, since adult ADHD is only in recent years becoming more recognized, it is reasonable to seek out services from an individual who has experience in the diagnosis and treatment of ADHD in that population. For many cases of ADHD, the treatment can be managed by a wide variety of clinicians as noted in Question 27. If, however, there is comorbidity with other psychiatric illness, or little or no response to traditional treatments, then it is reasonable to see someone more specialized, usually a psychiatrist. Even when seeing a psychiatrist, however, be sure the person you are seeing is comfortable and experienced with treating adult ADHD. The evaluation and treatment of this disorder has only recently been more emphasized in general psychiatry training programs; it has mainly been a part of the curriculum of child and adolescent psychiatry training programs. Child and adolescent psychiatrists may be a good choice for ADHD treatment of any age, because most child and adolescent psychiatrists treat adults as well.

Some individuals look specifically for a **psychopharmacologist**. The term can be somewhat misleading, as it implies a specialty in medication management of psychiatric conditions. In fact, all general psychiatrists are adequately trained in pharmacotherapy of mental disorders and need not be designated as psychopharmacologists. There is not a subspecialty

Treatment

Metabolize

The process of breaking down a drug in the blood.

QT interval

A measurement on electrocardiogram that represents the total duration of electrical activity of the ventricles of the heart; abnormal QT intervals may be evidence for increased risk of abnormal heart rhythms.

Serotonin syndrome

An extremely rare but life-threatening syndrome associated with the direct physiological effects of serotonin overload on the body. Symptoms include flushing, high fever, tachycardia, and seizures.

Psychopharmacologist

A specialist in the study of actions, effects, and development of psychoactive medications.

of psychiatry with this title. Some psychiatrists restrict their practice to medication management of mental disorders and are thus self-described as psychopharmacologists. They may tend to specialize in certain conditions and have unique expertise in the use of medications for more refractory cases, by virtue of clinical experience and perhaps research in academic settings. The specific subspecialties in the field of psychiatry are child and adolescent psychiatrists, geriatric psychiatrists, consultation–liaison psychiatrists (specializing in the treatment of the medically ill), addiction psychiatrists, and forensic psychiatrists. Depending upon your unique situation, one of these specialists may be needed.

64. How do stimulants for ADHD differ from illicit drugs like cocaine?

Cocaine is a stimulant with a chemical structure that is similar to that of methylphenidate and, like methylphenidate, it will raise alertness and productivity. Cocaine does so in the same fashion as methylphenidate, by increasing dopamine levels in the brain via blockade of dopamine reuptake. Cocaine, however, is a highly addictive drug ,which has led many to question whether methylphenidate and similar stimulants can lead to drug abuse. Key to the addictive potential of a drug is the speed with which it raises dopamine levels in the brain as well as the speed of clearance from the brain, rates that are quicker with cocaine than with methylphenidate. Oral methylphenidate takes one hour to raise dopamine levels while inhaled cocaine takes only seconds to do so. If a stimulant medication is ingested by a method other than prescribed, such as via inhalation, then its addictive potential will rise as well. This is how a stimulant medication might be abused. When crushed and snorted, thus increasing delivery to the brain, effects of stimulants are more akin to those of cocaine.

Key to the addictive potential of a drug is the speed with which it raises dopamine levels in the brain as well as the speed of clearance from the brain.

Rates of cocaine abuse are significantly higher in ADHD individuals than in the general population. It is thought possible that cocaine use serves as self-medication. Cocaine may help individuals with ADHD to focus and feel calm and in control, and indeed many adults who seek ADHD treatment report histories of cocaine abuse.

65. I have been prescribed a medication "off-label." Does that mean it is experimental?

The term **off-label** is used when a medication is used in a manner that is not FDA approved. Does this mean the medication is experimental? No, absolutely not. This means simply that no studies have been submitted to the FDA for approval of the medication for that particular use. It *does not mean* that no studies have been done. There are many studies on medications performed that are not submitted, or that have been submitted and approved by European governments. It *does not mean* that the medication is not widely prescribed for a use other than what the FDA approved. It *does not mean* that doses under or over the recommended range approved by the FDA are either ineffective or unsafe. And lastly, it *does not mean* that the medication is not safe in age groups younger or older than what the FDA approved. FDA approval merely means that when the company submitted the medication for approval, studies were submitted that specified a diagnosis, a dosage range, and an age group that the study subjects reflected.

Drug research and development has a fascinating history. Psychiatric drugs are often discovered serendipitously. Most drugs have multiple effects on the body, and focusing on one particular action to the exclusion of another is often as much a matter of marketing as it is drug action. For example, the first **antipsychotic** medication was developed and tested by a trauma surgeon who was specifically interested in finding a medication that could prevent surgical shock, a condition with a high mortality rate at the time. It was only through clinical observation that it was discovered to have antipsychotic effects as well as a variety of other effects on the body. The company that originally introduced it to the United States did not believe there would be a market for it as an antipsychotic and

Off-label

Prescribing of a medication for indications other than those outlined by the Food and Drug Administration.

Antipsychotic

A drug that treats psychotic symptoms, such as hallucinations, delusions, and thought disorders. Antipsychotics can be used to treat certain mood disorders as well.

so released it to the public as an anti-emetic. Only through multiple physician-driven lectures were psychiatrists in the United States comfortable enough to try it on patients suffering from schizophrenia. Perhaps even odder is the fact that the first antidepressant effects were observed in medications developed to treat tuberculosis. Dextroamphetamine came from amphetamine, which was first developed to treat cold symptoms, but was noticed to have effects on attention.

The group name of a medication, such as antidepressant, antipsychotic, or stimulant in actuality reflects the target population a particular medication is geared toward when released to the public, and not the broad range of effects of which the medication is capable. It also reflects the expense the companies go through in order to obtain FDA approval. The FDA requires that each medication target a specific diagnosis in order to receive approval. This is a hugely expensive enterprise for one diagnosis, much less for multiple diagnoses. Therefore, it is unlikely that drug companies will submit studies for approval for more than one or two diagnoses or for use in a different age group unless they can see some return on investment. As a result, clinical practice is often very different from what the *Physicians' Desk Reference* publishes. Clinical practice moves at a much faster pace than clinical trials and publications can keep up with. And while clinical trials are considered to be the definitive evidence of any particular medication's efficacy, astute clinical observations are what brought the biggest drug discoveries to the world and cannot be discounted simply because no study has yet to be published.

There are two broad reasons why off-label use makes sense in psychiatry. First, psychiatric diagnoses do not fit into the neat little categories the *DSM-IV-TR* attempts to define. They generally have many overlapping symptoms. It is recognized that ADHD is a result of dopamine and norepinephrine imbalances, and thus medications that affect these neurotransmitters, such as bupropion and venlafaxine, are utilized off-label as treatment options for ADHD. Many psychiatrists believe that medications should be prescribed to target the particular neurochemicals underlying such specific symptoms regardless of the DSM diagnosis. Off-label use is practiced with a clear rationale for another reason as well. Human nature defies categories. While there may be broad similarities between two individuals suffering from ADHD, it is doubtful that any one individual is suffering in exactly the same way as another from both a biochemical and psychological standpoint. Thus, one may respond to one particular therapy or medication and not another and the reasons are due to the therapies' and antidepressants' biochemical differences, not their similarities. For these reasons, off-label use in psychiatry is more the rule than the exception.

66. Are there benefits to taking "drug holidays?"

Associated with the use of stimulant medication is the notion of a "drug holiday." What is meant by this term is that the medication is purposely stopped for a period of time, such as during vacations, on weekends, or for entire summers. The phenomenon of stopping medication for these time periods is connected to treatment of children and adolescents with breaks from medication corresponding to school breaks and holidays. At one time ADHD was thought to be of concern mainly in the academic setting, and its treatment outside of classroom time was not widely practiced. The notion of taking the medication "for school" was common. As it became apparent within the medical community that ADHD affected all facets of a child's functioning, with areas outside of academics also being considered important for development, breaks from the medication became more discouraged.

Medication breaks were also encouraged in children and adolescents due to concerns of growth suppression. It is widely believed that when off stimulant medication, "catch-up" growth occurs. While some growth effects have been found in recent studies, the effects of "drug holidays" on growth have not been ascertained in controlled studies to date.

What this all means is that the notion of a "drug holiday" really has little meaning for adults. While doses of medication can be safely skipped, regularly doing so would likely diminish positive effects of the medication over time, because adults are usually seeking treatment due to problems with functioning across settings, none of which are regularly absent for a given time period. In the adult population, there is no benefit to be had by taking sustained breaks from the medication, unless you are specifically doing so to test a time period of functioning without medicine to see if you can get by without it.

While doses of medication can be safely skipped, regularly doing so would likely diminish positive effects of the medication over time.

Other medications used for ADHD should not be stopped for any period, because their effects are based upon stabilized blood levels achieved through regular, consistent dosing.

67. Can I drink wine with my ADHD medication?

Moderation should always be followed in drinking, but especially when under treatment with medication. For individuals with ADHD who are already at risk for impulsivity and over-indulgence in the use of alcohol, it is especially important to be cognizant of the adverse effects alcohol can have on attention and behavioral control. Stimulant medications can intensify the effects of alcohol, making inebriation more likely with lesser amounts of alcohol than when not taking medication. It is best to limit alcohol intake to no more than one or two drinks. You can skip your stimulant medication for the day (with long-acting medication, this may not be possible unless planned for earlier), but this is not a useful long-term strategy, nor does it work for medications that must be taken daily. Also, consider the impact that skipping your medication will have on your functioning for the day. A few extra drinks in the evening may not be worth the day of disorganization and the complications that can come with it.

With antidepressant medications used for ADHD, the risks of use in combination with alcohol are due to their sedative effects, which are additive to alcohol, and thus more readily cause intoxication and its incumbent risks. This effect may be more likely with TCAs than with the SSRIs, because these medications are not found to be sedating or adversely affecting cognition and motor coordination. While on an antidepressant, it is best to be cautious in monitoring its effect on your mental status if having wine or other alcohol.

68. How does generic medication differ from brand name medication?

The generic name of a medication is the international scientific name for the molecule that constitutes the active form of the medication. The company that develops the medication then applies for a patent and obtains exclusive rights to sell the medication. They then give the medication a brand, or trade, name. This brand name can change from country to country and from its intended use. For example, the medication with the generic name paroxetine is marketed under the trade name Paxil in the United States and Seroxat in the United Kingdom. The medication with the generic name bupropion is used as an antidepressant under the trade name Wellbutrin and as a smoking cessation medication under the name Zyban. The medication with the generic name fluoxetine is used under the trade name Prozac as an antidepressant and as Sarafem, a medication prescribed by obstetricians, for women suffering from premenstrual symptoms. Once a medication goes off patent, other companies obtain the right to make it and sell it. At this point, generic forms of the medication that may be less expensive become available. These medications are sold under their generic names. As physicians first know the original form of the medication by its trade name, they often continue to write prescriptions under that name. By law, pharmacies must fill the prescription with the less expensive form of the medication unless the physician specifically indicates to the pharmacy not to substitute. As a result, the filled prescription will come back to the patient under the generic name rather than the trade name.

The generic name of a medication is the international scientific name for the molecule that constitutes the active form of the medication.

Are there differences between generic medications and medications under the trade name? The active ingredients of the medication are identical. The "fillers" or inactive ingredients making up the rest of the medication may differ. There may also be more percentage variations between the amounts of active ingredients from pill to pill in generic medications than in trade medications as the requirements for quantity control are more stringent with trade medications than with generic medications. These differences are so minute as to be negligible for most individuals, particularly for medications that work over time, but in cases of stimulants that work on a day-to-day basis, it is possible to notice a difference if particularly sensitive to the medication being taken. If available in generic, it is not unreasonable to try the generic medication first due to the considerable cost savings.

69. What if my spouse doesn't want to get treatment for ADHD?

It can be difficult for the non-ADHD spouse or partner to live with someone who exhibits significant problems related to attention and impulse control. It can be easy to assume your partner is being passive aggressive or lazy when he or she is procrastinating or forgetful. It is important to keep in mind that the individual with ADHD may be impaired and unable to perform at the expected level of functioning. Resentment, anger, criticism, and judgment can often create friction in marriages and partnerships. Insight into the nature of ADHD as an illness can make it less frustrating for partners to deal with their ADHD partners. If, however, the ADHD partner refuses to be evaluated or treated, the situation can become even more frustrating. Perhaps your partner is biased against psychiatry and is afraid of being labeled or of taking medication. Sometimes it can be helpful if the couple's child is in treatment for ADHD. When parents see improvement in their child, it is easier to think about the possibility of improvement for them too. You can try providing your partner with information from the Internet or from books regarding the illness. For you, there are books about living with family members with ADHD that can be helpful. If your partner is still reluctant to enter into treatment, consider asking him or her to enter couples therapy to address communication problems. In this way, your partner can better see how his or her behavior impacts the relationship, and you can learn how your responses affect your partner. Once communication is better facilitated in this way, your partner may eventually opt to be evaluated for his or her condition.

70. Are ADHD medications prescribed for other conditions?

As noted in an earlier question, many psychotropic medications are utilized for reasons other than the FDA-approved use. Stimulants, however, are used primarily for the treatment of ADHD. Both dextroamphetamine and methylphenidate have indications for narcolepsy as well. Methylphenidate may be utilized for **augmentation** in the treatment of depression and may be used for cognitive impairment secondary to traumatic brain injury; however, these are considered off-label uses. Amphetamines were previously used in the treatment of obesity; however, they are no longer utilized in that capacity.

Augmentation

In pharmacotherapy, a strategy of using a second medication to enhance the positive effects of an existing medication in the regimen.

Atomoxetine is being studied for its utility in the treatment of depression because it is a norepinephrine reuptake inhibitor with a mechanism of action similar to some antidepressants. While not prescribed as a primary treatment for depression, it is often prescribed for ADHD in the presence of comorbid depression or anxiety in an effort to use one medication to treat both conditions.

Both bupropion and venlafaxine are antidepressants used primarily to treat depression and/or anxiety disorders. Their use in the treatment of ADHD is off-label. Clonidine and guanfacine are off-label ADHD medications that have indications as anti-hypertensive agents, and modafinil is indicated for treatment of narcolepsy.

PART FIVE

Associated Conditions

What conditions are commonly associated
with ADHD?

I have been diagnosed with depression and ADHD.
How is the combination of conditions treated?

Can ADHD be associated with a lot of panic
and worrying?

More . . .

71. What conditions are commonly associated with ADHD?

Additional psychiatric disorders in the presence of ADHD occur at rates as high as 50% to 75%. The most common comorbid conditions are Major Depressive Disorder, Generalized Anxiety Disorder, Bipolar Disorder, and substance abuse. Antisocial Personality Disorder is common as well. Antisocial Personality Disorder is more likely to occur when childhood ADHD is comorbid with Oppositional Defiant Disorder followed by Conduct Disorder, both of which are disruptive behavioral disorders diagnosed in childhood and adolescence. Conduct Disorder is characterized by criminal behaviors that can persist into adulthood.

Oftentimes, adults present with symptoms of a comorbid disorder as the initial complaint, unaware that ADHD may be a significant factor in the symptom picture as well.

Oftentimes, adults present with symptoms of a comorbid disorder as the initial complaint, unaware that ADHD may be a significant factor in the symptom picture as well. When ADHD is discovered upon evaluation, the clinician needs to determine which disorder is the primary source of the presenting complaints and which should be treated first. It is often the case that with treatment of ADHD, depressive or anxiety disorders can improve markedly. This may be due to the fact that the depressive or anxious symptoms are driven by the repeated frustrations and limitations that occur on a daily basis in the presence of ADHD. Also possible, however, is that the comorbid depressive or anxiety disorder exacerbates the ADHD, making its symptoms worse. For these reasons, it is usually better to attempt to treat one condition at a time. If there is no improvement in one condition with traditional treatments, it may be reasonable to go ahead and treat the other; an untreated comorbid condition can render traditional treatments less effective.

72. I have been diagnosed with depression and ADHD. How is the combination of conditions treated?

Part of a complete evaluation for ADHD includes an evaluation for other conditions that may be a cause for the attention symptoms or that may be concurrent with a diagnosis of ADHD. If other conditions are determined to be comorbid with the ADHD, a decision as to how those conditions should be treated is made as well. Rates of depression are high in adults with ADHD, with a prevalence rate of major depression two times greater than in the general population. In reverse, rates of ADHD in adults with major depression are also at a higher prevalence rate than ADHD in adults without major depression. The two disorders can usually be readily distinguished as they share only two symptoms: diminished concentration or attention and **psychomotor agitation**.

Depending upon the severity of the depression, it may or may not need to be treated prior to initiating pharmacotherapy for ADHD. Depression may occur secondary to untreated ADHD, so if the depression is judged to be mild, treatment of the ADHD may result in remission of depressive symptoms. Mild major depression or dysthymia may have developed as a result of the complications of living with untreated ADHD. Problems in work and relationships commonly occur with untreated ADHD, both of which can be stressors that trigger depression. In addition, self-esteem is frequently adversely affected due to frequent negative feedback during interactions with others. If the depression is moderate to severe, and especially if suicidal ideation is present, then treatment of the depression should be undertaken first. Once stabilized, ADHD symptoms may not be as severe because depression adversely effects concentration. Also, treatment with a stimulant medication is not as likely to exacerbate the depressive or even anxious symptoms, which can sometimes occur as a side effect to stimulant medications. In treating the depression first, your doctor may opt to use one of the antidepressants also used off-label to treat ADHD, such as bupropion or venlafaxine; however, other antidepressants may be used if considered more clinically appropriate. Once stabilized, stimulants can be safely taken with most antidepressant medications (except the monoamine oxidase inhibitors), as can atomoxetine or the antihypertensive medications.

Associated Conditions

Psychomotor agitation

Hyperactive or restless movement. It can be seen in highly anxious states, manic mood states, or intoxicated states.

While not always necessary for the treatment of ADHD alone, psychotherapy is an important component of treatment for depression with ADHD. With psychotherapy, medication may not be required to treat the depressive disorder, and if cognitive behavioral therapy is utilized, it can be used to address management of ADHD symptoms as well.

73. Can ADHD be associated with a lot of panic and worrying?

Anxiety disorders are frequently comorbid with ADHD, including Obsessive-Compulsive Disorder (OCD), Social Phobia, Generalized Anxiety Disorder (GAD), and Panic Disorder. Anywhere from 25% to 40% of adults with ADHD also have an anxiety disorder. Rates of specific anxiety disorders are higher in ADHD adults than in the general population. This can be due to independent risks for each condition, or due to combined effects. Note also that there is a higher rate of ADHD among adults with anxiety disorders than among those without anxiety, although the rate of anxiety in ADHD adults is far greater than the rate of ADHD in anxiety disorder adults. Certainly, anxiety levels can be heightened in the presence of ADHD, due to the difficulty in keeping up with responsibilities and the potentially negative effects at home and in the workplace. So while the development of anxiety disorders in persons with ADHD could be due to separate genetic effects, they may also arise secondarily as a result of living with ADHD symptoms. With this in mind, it has been theorized that treatment of ADHD in childhood could potentially prevent later onset of anxiety and depressive disorders. It can be difficult to ascertain whether the ADHD or anxiety is the more severe condition for a given individual, but the presence of anxiety can significantly exacerbate ADHD symptoms and ADHD can exacerbate anxiety. In the presence of a feeling of being overwhelmed, panic attacks can occur. Poor concentration and restlessness are characteristic of GAD as well as ADHD. Fear of acting on impulse can result in social avoidance. Compulsions of OCD can often offset the disorganization that can occur with ADHD, which can make it difficult to identify ADHD symptoms in these cases. Due to the significant rates of comorbidity, it is important that adults with ADHD and those with anxiety disorders be evaluated for both conditions.

74. My anxiety became worse when I took a stimulant for ADHD. What can I do?

ADHD can be successfully treated in the presence of an anxiety disorder; however, management becomes more complex and should probably be undertaken by a psychiatrist who specializes in the treatment of ADHD. Protocols for treating ADHD in the presence of anxiety depend somewhat upon the severity of the anxious symptoms. This is why it is important to have a full diagnostic evaluation to assess for the presence of a significant anxiety disorder. Stimulants can worsen underlying anxiety symptoms, for example, by exacerbating the worrying in GAD or by increasing obsessions and compulsions in OCD. If anxiety occurs as a result of untreated ADHD symptoms, a stimulant may actually reduce the anxiety. Sometimes it is unclear whether the anxiety disorder is a separate entity, but a reasonable approach can be to try a stimulant first because this medication is easily started and stopped without a long period of medication withdrawal. If the anxiety is in fact worsened, then treatment of the anxiety will be needed in order to successfully treat the ADHD. One option is to use atomoxetine to treat the ADHD without risk of exacerbating the anxiety, which may also treat the anxiety. If the anxiety disorder is severe and a medication shown to treat it is desired, then use of venlafaxine to treat the anxiety might be considered with the possibility it will also treat the ADHD. Alternatively, if an SSRI is thought necessary, such as for OCD, then it can be prescribed first for the anxiety disorder and, once those symptoms are under control, a stimulant can be added to treat the ADHD. These are just some of the possible approaches that your physician can go over with you. Again, which approach is best will depend upon the specific anxiety disorder and its severity.

In the presence of a comorbid anxiety disorder, adjunctive psychotherapy such as cognitive behavioral therapy is a good idea to facilitate response to the pharmacologic treatment. If the anxiety disorder is mild in degree, psychotherapy may provide enough of an intervention so that medication is needed for ADHD alone.

75. How are alcoholism and ADHD connected?

The presentation of comorbid substance abuse disorders and ADHD is common, and research has shown high rates of ADHD in substance abusers in addition to ADHD being a risk factor for substance abuse.

The presentation of comorbid substance abuse disorders and ADHD is common, and research has shown high rates of ADHD in substance abusers in addition to ADHD being a risk factor for substance abuse. Approximately half of adults who report ADHD symptoms also report a coexisting substance abuse disorder. Individuals with ADHD have a higher risk for both alcohol and drug abuse. Prevalence of ADHD in the substance abusing population is from 15% to 25%. Adults with ADHD start abusing substances at an earlier age and abuse substances more often than those without ADHD. They are also more likely to move more quickly past alcohol to other substances.

Factors associated with the highest risk for substance use disorders in ADHD patients include disruptive behavior disorders, Bipolar Disorder, eating disorders, low socioeconomic status, and dropping out of school. In addition to core ADHD symptoms facilitating the risk for substance use disorders, the sequelae of poorly-controlled ADHD may contribute to the development of substance abuse. The mean age of onset of substance abuse in ADHD adults is earlier than the mean age for non-ADHD adults. Adults with ADHD are more likely to progress from an alcohol use disorder to a drug use disorder then non-ADHD adults and have greater difficulty maintaining remission.

76. My spouse is drinking a lot of alcohol lately. My friend thinks he might be self-medicating. What does that mean?

Alcoholism is present in higher percentages of individuals with ADHD than in the general population. Individuals with anxiety, **mood disorders**, or even ADHD may abuse alcohol or drugs in a misguided effort to feel better. Depression is common in the presence of ADHD, and the transient improvement in mood that comes with alcohol consumption can facilitate its abuse; however, over the long term, alcohol is actually a depressant. Likewise, use of drugs to get "high" is usually followed by a "crash" during which the mood becomes sad or despondent. Sometimes alcohol or drug abuse itself will cause the depression, which will remit when abstinence is achieved. Oftentimes, depression precedes the alcohol or drug use, and people turn to these substances in an effort to feel better. Typically, though, feeling better really just means being "numb" or deadened to the depressed feelings. Treatment of the depression may result in achievement of abstinence. This of course will depend on the stage of substance abuse. If the individual has become dependent upon/addicted to the alcohol or drugs, then concordant substance abuse treatment will likely be necessary as well. As long as the person is addicted to alcohol or drugs, recovery from depression will be limited. In fact, substance abuse is a problem that needs to be considered if someone is refractory to treatments for depression, ADHD, or other conditions. Seeing a person who specializes in treatment of addictions would also be helpful because different forms of therapeutic interventions are often needed in persons who have addiction. In addition, there are specialized treatment programs for persons with both mental illness and substance abuse. The self-medication hypothesis would assume the drug of choice acts in a way that is similar to medications that treat ADHD. Alcohol would not be considered to act in a similar fashion; however, the "self-medicating" aspect of its use may be connected to its mood altering effects.

Mood disorder

A type of mental illness that affects mood primarily and cognition secondarily. Mood disorders predominantly consist of depression and bipolar disorder.

Associated Conditions

77. If substance abuse is a risk of untreated ADHD, why am I being asked to have drug treatment first? Can't I receive ADHD treatment first?

Patients with a combination of addiction and ADHD are at higher risk for mood disorders, along with suicide, homicide, poor compliance, and relapse. While there is some evidence to support the concept that many patients use substances to "self-medicate" underlying symptoms, there is no evidence that treatment with a stimulant or nonstimulant leads to abstinence. In fact, both medication groups have the contraindication of prescribing in the presence of active substance abuse. Stimulants have the contraindication of prescribing in the presence of a history of substance abuse as well. While these contraindications are considered "relative," meaning that individual circumstances can be taken into account by the clinician, they do highlight the fact that use of ADHD medications with active substance abuse poses various risks. One risk, of course, is that the medication will be used as a substance of abuse. Another risk is the potential for complications secondary to the combination of drugs and medications, such as death due to cardiac arrest. While the "self-medication hypothesis" may seem right for some individuals, once an addiction develops it takes on a life of its own. It is unlikely that medicating it away can conquer addiction. Also, if you continue to use drugs or alcohol while receiving treatment for your ADHD, you essentially render the treatment ineffective. Thus, in the presence of addiction, ADHD cannot be effectively treated without also treating the addiction. Once the addiction is in remission, various treatment approaches for the ADHD can be considered. However linked they may have been in their origins, they are now separate entities, and both require treatment in order for you to return to health.

78. Can ADHD be treated before remission of substance abuse?

The use of stimulants in the presence of active substance abuse is labeled by the FDA as a contraindication, and the typical treatment course that is recommended is to treat the substance use disorder first, then address the ADHD once substance abuse is in remission (Question 77). The problem with this approach, however, is that substance use disorders tend to be worse in ADHD adults, so the risk for relapse of the substance use disorder in the absence of ADHD treatment is higher. That said, the risk for substance abuse in the presence of ADHD is high, and some argue that treatment of the ADHD would likely mitigate the substance abuse.

One of the potential problems with initiating ADHD treatment prior to remission of substance abuse is that it can be difficult to diagnose ADHD in the presence of active substance abuse. This is generally considered to be the case for most psychiatric disorders because substances of abuse are to be excluded as the cause of the symptoms. It is possible, with a careful assessment that includes thorough history in the absence of substance use, to diagnose a comorbid disorder such as ADHD. Some studies have looked at the use of stimulants to treat ADHD while patients are in substance abuse treatment. In a 2002 study by Schubiner et al., methylphenidate was safely given to a group of cocaine-abusing adults; but, while there was a reduction in ADHD symptoms, there was no reduction in cocaine use. At present, the contraindication to use of stimulants in the presence of active substance use is due to the potential increased cardiovascular risk, particularly with abuse of a **sympathomimetic** drug such as cocaine. Atomoxetine also carries a similar warning, so caution would be required in the treatment of ADHD during active substance abuse.

Sympathomimetic

Mimics the effects of stimulation of organs and structures by the sympathetic nervous system.

79. Is there a connection between cigarette smoking and ADHD?

There is a high correlation between nicotine addiction and psychiatric disorders, including ADHD.

There is a high correlation between nicotine addiction and psychiatric disorders, including ADHD. The rate of smoking in ADHD adults is approximately 40% in comparison to a rate of about 25% in non-ADHD adults. Rates of nicotine addiction are also higher in ADHD adolescents in comparison to non-ADHD adolescents. Individuals with ADHD have reported earlier initiation of smoking and greater difficulty in quitting as well.

Many studies indicate that core ADHD symptoms confer a risk for smoking, even in the absence of a clinical diagnosis of ADHD. In other words, symptoms along the inattentive domain and the hyperactive-impulsive domain have shown associations with various smoking-related behaviors. Some studies have shown a stronger association between hyperactivity and impulsivity with smoking than the inattentive subtype.

What is known about smoking in the general population is that the earlier the initiation of smoking, the greater the likelihood of addiction and the greater the difficulty in quitting, such that the risk-taking behavior characteristic of the hyperactive-impulsive type of ADHD may confer a greater risk for earlier experimentation, and thus later addiction. In terms of nicotine dependence and subsequent difficulty in quitting, it is considered a possibility that attention and focus are improved by nicotine use. Current research is examining the connection between attention and nicotinic receptors in the brain.

Liza comments,

I smoked cigarettes from my junior year in high school through my sophomore year in college. It was extremely difficult to quit. Cigarettes calmed me down and I became a habitual smoker very quickly. I can never be "a social smoker." I never want to have to quit again.

80. *Is there an overlap between ADHD and bipolar disorder?*

The prevalence of ADHD and bipolar disorder co-occurring in adults is high, with rates in studies found to range from approximately 9% to 21% of bipolar adults having ADHD, with bipolar disorder occurring in approximately 19% of adults with ADHD. In the presence of ADHD, bipolar individuals have higher rates of manic episodes, suicide attempts, violence, and legal problems. The coexistence of the two conditions may be related to the age of onset of bipolar disorder, as adults with a reported history of comorbid ADHD tend to have the onset of bipolar disorder before age 19. Studies of rates of ADHD in the children of bipolar adults have found higher rates than in control subjects. It has been argued that ADHD is misdiagnosed in some young people who actually have bipolar disorder, although a high number of youth with bipolar disorder also have ADHD.

While ADHD is a condition distinct from bipolar disorder, the differentiation of mania from ADHD can be difficult. There are similarities in symptoms, particularly in the presentation of children and adolescents. Both disorders share many characteristics such as impulsivity, inattention, hyperactivity, high physical energy, mood swings, frequent coexistence of conduct disorder and oppositional-defiant disorder, and learning problems. Family history in both conditions often has the presence of mood disorders. Enduring elevated mood and grandiosity are the symptoms best able to distinguish between bipolar disorder and ADHD. Also, with bipolar disorder, symptoms in general tend to be episodic in contrast to the pervasiveness of symptoms due to ADHD. Irritability, hyperactivity, accelerated speech, and distractibility are frequent in both bipolar disorder and ADHD and are not useful in differentiating between the two disorders. The response or lack of response to stimulant medications is not diagnostically helpful, but classification of the diagnosis is important as stimulants may promote mania

Mood stabilizer

Typically refers to medications used for the treatment and prevention of mood swings, such as those from depression and mania.

in a bipolar individual if not on a **mood stabilizer** first (as with antidepressants).

81. How are bipolar disorder and ADHD treated together?

In the presence of bipolar disorder, it is important to treat active bipolar symptoms before treating the ADHD. ADHD symptoms are not likely to resolve in the presence of active bipolar symptoms, and stimulants used for ADHD are thought potentially contributory to mood swings in bipolar individuals. Once the mood is stabilized, the ADHD symptoms can be reassessed. The severity of the symptoms may have resolved. If still present, a decision as to the best therapeutic approach needs to be made, keeping in mind the risk of triggering mania with the medication. While stimulants have been thought possibly contributory to mania in a bipolar individual, there is controversy regarding this theory due to an absence of supportive scientific evidence, so in the presence of a mood stabilizer, it would likely be safe to have a stimulant trial under your doctor's close monitoring. Atomoxetine may be more risky because of its similar chemical profile to antidepressants that are also considered potentially mania-inducing in the bipolar individual. Bupropion has been associated with less mood instability in comparison to other antidepressants, so this could be a considered intervention, particularly with **bipolar depression** in the presence of ADHD; however, this too has been shown to be associated with risk of switching from depression to mania, and should be used with a mood stabilizer on board as well.

Bipolar depression

An episode of depression that occurs in the course of bipolar disorder.

Psychotherapy can help facilitate remission and is a helpful adjunct in the treatment plan of bipolar patients. A cognitive-behavioral approach can also be utilized to address the ADHD symptoms.

82. How are learning disabilities and ADHD connected?

While ADHD and learning disabilities often occur together, they are not the same thing. Learning disabilities are neurological disorders that occur due to a deficit in the brain that affects processing of information. About 15% of Americans have some type of learning disability with 80% of those having reading problems. Learning disabilities often run in families. Learning disabilities have nothing to do with intellectual functioning or how "smart" someone is, much as ADHD has nothing to do with intelligence. Part of the differential in evaluating a child or adolescent for ADHD is consideration of a learning disability as the cause for any symptoms as children with learning disabilities may be restless or easily distracted. Of children with ADHD, 20% to 30% also have a learning disability. Keep in mind, too, that learning disabilities are lifelong as well. ADHD symptoms can resolve with treatment, whereas learning disabilities cannot. New ways of taking in information are usually needed in order to work around the disabilities.

While ADHD and learning disabilities often occur together, they are not the same thing.

Psychological testing can be helpful when it is unclear whether or not learning disabilities are present with the ADHD or if the symptoms are driven by undiagnosed learning disabilities. In identifying specific weaknesses, various methods of working around those weaknesses as well as developing strengths can be recommended.

83. How are ADHD and Tourette's syndrome connected?

Tourette's syndrome is a disorder characterized by various motor and/or vocal tics, such as eye blinks, facial twitches, grimacing, frequent throat clearing, snorting, sniffing, or barking out words. Tourette's syndrome is a more severe form of tic disorders, the most common being a simple tic disorder characterized by a single tic such as eye blinking or throat clearing. While very few children have Tourette's syndrome,

Associated Conditions

many who have Tourette's syndrome have associated ADHD, with comorbidity reported to be as high as 90%. While only a small proportion of people with ADHD have Tourette's syndrome, the presence of tics without full blown Tourette's syndrome is relatively common in children with ADHD. The onset of ADHD and tic disorders tends to occur around the same age, with tics and Tourette's syndrome thought to occur in as many as 50% of children diagnosed with ADHD. While simple tic disorders may not necessitate treatment, those with multiple tics or Tourette's are likely to require treatment. Treatment of tics is with medication, and in the presence of ADHD it may be possible to treat both conditions with one medication, as clonidine and guanfacine are helpful in reducing tic frequency and severity. Stimulant treatment for ADHD can in some cases exacerbate tics; however, the presence of tics is not considered an absolute contraindication to use of stimulants by clinicians who work with Tourette's patients. If the tics are treated, they may not be exacerbated with the use of stimulants. Atomoxetine is a medication of choice when there is concern for possibly exacerbating tics because it has not been found to do so.

84. Is there a connection between eating disorders and ADHD?

The risk for development of eating disorders in girls with ADHD is an under-recognized problem. A recent longitudinal study found that girls with ADHD were more likely to develop an eating disorder than girls without ADHD. Eating disorders are more common in girls than in boys, so this may be a risk factor of ADHD that is greater in girls than in boys. Eating disorders tend to develop in adolescence but often persist into adulthood, so adults with ADHD may have a concurrent or history of an eating disorder. In one study, the risk was greater for bulimic disorders than for anorexia nervosa, although both conditions were of heightened risk. In a later study, findings were similar for risk. Girls with combined-type ADHD were the most likely to have bulimic disorders in contrast to both the inattentive subtype girls and controls. Girls from both ADHD subtypes were more likely to be overweight, as well as to have been subjected to critical parents and peer rejection at greater rates than girls without ADHD. It was postulated from those results that those psychosocial factors may have contributed to the onset of the eating disorders. While the causes of eating disorders are multifactorial with genetic, familial, and psychological factors contributing, certainly symptoms of ADHD could increase the susceptibility in combination with other factors due to the negative impact ADHD symptoms can have on family dynamics and on self-esteem.

As opposed to development of anorexic and bulimic disorders, the impulsivity from ADHD can extend to eating patterns as well, with many ADHD adults engaging in overeating or disordered eating, which can result in obesity. Many adults with ADHD report compulsively overeating, often in an effort to relieve stress and induce calm. Problems with self-control and regulation can affect food choices and patterns of eating. To begin with, lack of planning and running behind make you susceptible to eating food on the go, which is not likely to be healthy food. In addition, erratic eating schedules, such as late in the evening, can result in excessive overeating. Some people with ADHD find they crave carbohydrates and sweet foods. They may be more apt to eat due to boredom, anger, or sadness as well as for self-stimulation, as a reward, and for stress relief. Food can have a calming effect when feeling overwhelmed and stressed, problems that are common for adults with ADHD. Treatment for ADHD may help with developing better eating patterns, but a plan would need to be put in place to facilitate the change.

Samantha comments,

I was diagnosed with ADHD when I was 45 years old. I had an eating disorder for over thirty years prior to that. Medications had been prescribed to help me with my eating disorder (bulimia). When my ADHD was treated with stimulants my eating disorder immediately went into remission. There are days I fail to take my

ADHD medication and the urge to engage in binging and purging resurfaces. Research that I have read does indicate that stimulants can be effective for some types of eating disorders, but this research is very new.

85. Is there a link between creativity and ADHD?

Many people with ADHD excel at thinking outside of the box, brainstorming, and finding creative solutions to problems. Their ability to hyperfocus may enable them to solve problems in a unique way. Common traits are open-mindedness and independence. Many well-known creative individuals are believed to have ADHD. Some of the traits often described to occur in highly creative individuals are:

- Inattention
- Daydreaming
- Inability to complete projects
- Hyperactivity
- Moodiness
- Difficult temperament
- Social skills deficits
- Sensation seeking

As can be seen from the list, there is significant overlap with ADHD symptoms. It is argued, however, that some highly creative individuals do not have ADHD and some individuals with ADHD are not creative. Many people with ADHD also have creativity, and the two do not have to be mutually exclusive. Perhaps the traits of ADHD allow for enhanced creativity. Or perhaps there is a similar underlying mechanism. Regardless, there is no reason the two cannot exist together.

Sometimes individuals who undergo creative work will find that it is more difficult to work in the same way with their medication on board. If this is the case, the medication can possibly be reduced or prescribed for a shorter duration of the day.

86. Is it possible to have ADHD and a high IQ?

Intellectual functioning has no correlation to the development of ADHD, although either low or high IQ may impede the recognition of ADHD. Due to the presence of learning difficulties associated with a lower IQ, however, such an individual is more apt to come to clinical attention and thus be found to have co-occurring ADHD than an individual with a high IQ. It is often the case that such children and adolescents do not come to clinical attention because they are able to develop compensatory strategies for dealing with ADHD symptoms. High scores in the classroom may come easily to them, and thus they are not identified as having difficulties. Perhaps the child gets all Bs and is told simply that he or she can do better. There may be subtle complaints such as talking too much or daydreaming made by the teachers, but as long as grades are kept up, neither parents nor teachers are apt to consider that a problem may exist. Difficulties may not occur academically until high school or college, when work demands increase and when more independence in studying is required. In studies on ADHD adults with high IQ, many had dropped out of postsecondary education or were under- or unemployed. On neuropsychological testing, scores on tests related to attention and concentration tend to be impaired in relation to intelligence scores. Studies of ADHD youth with high IQs have also supported its existence and have found higher rates of mood, anxious, and disruptive behavior disorders in high IQ youth with ADHD in contrast to those without ADHD.

Intellectual functioning has no correlation to the development of ADHD, although either low or high IQ may impede the recognition of ADHD.

Associated Conditions

PART SIX

Living with ADHD

How can I manage my life with ADHD?

What are issues faced by women with ADHD?

How can I succeed in college with ADHD?

More . . .

87. *How can I manage my life with ADHD?*

While people do not usually outgrow ADHD, they do learn to adapt. Learning how to manage symptoms throughout life will enable you to use your personal strengths to grow and be successful. You can utilize various strategies to help manage ADHD on a daily basis such as:

- Taking medications as directed
- Organizing yourself
- Learning to control impulsive behavior
- Minimizing distractions
- Finding constructive outlets for excess energy
- Asking for help

Recognize your strengths rather than focusing on your weaknesses, and develop strategies for working around those weaknesses.

Recognize your strengths rather than focusing on your weaknesses, and develop strategies for working around those weaknesses. Look into various forms of psychosocial interventions such as individual therapy, coaching, organizational assistance, meditation, etc., that can help support your efforts to adapt and cope with your symptoms. Use of adjunctive strategies goes a long way in facilitating improvements in combination with medication.

Samantha comments,

Having ADHD does require me to do "additional work" to stay on task. Over many years of practice, however, I learned many ways to manage my symptoms. When in school and college I was still able to achieve high honors and then obtain work. In fact, I have always worked in demanding jobs. My motivation to be successful in educational and vocational pursuits took both time and dedication. Currently, I am engaged in the practice of mindfulness meditation. It has taken over a decade to achieve this practice, but it is very helpful to me as I continue to work at being focused and present.

Liza comments,

I have found things that work for me. Right now I am doing well on my medication. Medicine helps me focus. The routines I have, the

*process for doing things, work schedules, class schedules, radar detec-
tors, agenda books, lists for everything, sleep management, not carrying cash, using a debit card for everything, giving myself "time
outs" when I become too emotional and upset, sitting in the front
row when I have to pay attention, limiting my alcohol consumption,
and asking for help when I need it are some of the things I have
incorporated in my life. Medication alone did not fix my problems.
I am always working toward making my life a happy one.*

88. What are issues faced by women with ADHD?

In children and adolescents, ADHD is diagnosed more frequently in boys than in girls at close to a 4:1 ratio. This ratio
actually becomes 1:1 by adulthood however, and it is thought
likely that the gender discrepancy in childhood is due to the
fact that girls with ADHD are less likely to be recognized
and referred for treatment. One consideration is that girls
are thought to more likely have the inattentive subtype of
ADHD over the hyperactive-impulsive subtype. Hyperactive
and impulsive children are more likely to come to the attention of healthcare professionals, while children who are inattentive (boys and girls) may "slip through the cracks" as they
are not overtly disruptive. Also, when hyperactive, girls are
more likely to exhibit their hyperactivity via excessive talking
or "chattiness" rather than running and climbing excessively.
Girls with ADHD are 5 times more likely to develop depression than girls without ADHD, and the depression is often
more severe and lasts longer. By adulthood, many women with
ADHD may be seeking treatment for depression, but have
unrecognized ADHD. In terms of ADHD symptoms as well,
in adulthood the predominant symptoms of concern for both
men and women are those secondary to inattentive features
of ADHD. As adults are self-referred, women are more apt
to seek treatment at this stage in their lives.

Unique issues faced by women include balancing of family
life with work and/or school demands. As women in society
today continue to be more involved than men in household
management and child rearing, women with ADHD face

unique challenges in these areas. Working mothers in particular may find that once-manageable symptoms become quickly consuming of their time and energy. Many women with ADHD feel unable to have guests in their homes due to the piles of clothes, papers, and other items strewn about the house. Household tasks and chores become overwhelming. They may yell frequently at their children due to low frustration tolerance and difficulty with multitasking. They may have difficulty setting limits and providing structure for their children, which can exacerbate relationship conflicts. Children in the household are also at a higher risk for developing ADHD, making the task of child rearing even more complicated. The risk for child abuse in the home increases, likely due to temper difficulties and impulsivity in affected parents.

Hormonal

Referring to the chemicals that are secreted by the endocrine glands (the thyroid, pancreas, pituitary glands, and others) and act throughout the body.

Additional issues faced by women center around **hormonal** changes that can have effects upon ADHD symptoms. When girls enter puberty, there can be notable changes in mood that can affect their ADHD symptoms. For many women, mood worsens premenstrually and can be exacerbated under the stress of ADHD symptoms. Estrogen levels impact mood, mental states, and memory. Studies in women have shown that estrogen improves memory and cognitive functioning. During perimenopause, in addition to mood changes, many women exhibit cognitive deficits. Both of these conditions can markedly worsen ADHD symptoms and may necessitate treatment adjustments.

Samantha comments,

I have always been more successful at work than I am at home. My problems with organization and staying focused and difficulty with sustaining my attention does impair my ability to be a "super-mom" or live in a "Donna Reed" world. At work, in the presence of structure, it was always easier to get things accomplished. At home with an active family life, there are a million and one things to do and I have to constantly prioritize. I desire organization, a very clean home, many hours to spend with my kids, time for friends and creating "perfect" social events, along with cooking, shopping, and exercise. Settling into "a few tasks" is difficult and accomplishing all that I desire is impossible, especially when working full time. It is essential that my husband "schedule" time for us. It is important that I am mindful of the importance of our quality time.

89. What can I do about my ADHD while pregnant and nursing?

An issue also unique to women is the management of ADHD both during and after pregnancy. At present, there is no adequate data to suggest whether any medications useful for ADHD are safe to use in pregnancy. All medications typically used for ADHD are classified under pregnancy category C, which basically means that those medications have not been shown to be harmful to a fetus, but the lack of data about their effects on fetal development would raise concern. Some animal studies have shown an increase in birth defects with the use of amphetamines. Low birth weight and higher pregnancy complications have been associated with amphetamines as well, although some of those studies were of substance abusing populations. Case reports on women exposed to methylphenidate during pregnancy have found higher than expected rates of prematurity, growth retardation, and neonatal medication withdrawal in the infants. Given these findings and lack of sufficient data, it would be best to work on nonpharmacologic interventions for dealing with ADHD during pregnancy. It is also possible that ADHD symptoms will reduce in intensity during the pregnancy, as higher estrogen levels are associated with better memory and other cognitive functions.

While breastfeeding, estrogen levels remain high, and thus ADHD symptoms are often reduced in intensity at this time. This may not hold true for everyone, however, and it can be frustrating to manage ADHD symptoms as a new mother. As the levels of ADHD medication found in breast milk are not known, it is generally advised that these medications not be taken while breastfeeding. If your circumstances are such that it remains difficult to stay off medications while breastfeeding, discuss your options with your doctor. You will have to weigh the risk of medication exposure against the benefits of breast milk over formula. Some women will utilize short-acting stimulant agents and pump and discard the milk while the medication is in their system. In theory, once the medication has been metabolized from your body, it would no longer enter the breast milk. As everyone metabolizes medications at differing rates, however, it would not be clear for a given person what stimulant levels, if any, would be present in the breast milk at a given time. These would be issues to discuss in greater detail with your doctor.

90. How can I succeed in college with ADHD?

Entering college can be a challenge for the young adult with ADHD, not simply due to the academic difficulties that can occur as a result of the symptoms, but also due to the new independence and higher level of responsibility. It is likely that a child with ADHD has been closely supervised and assisted by one or both parents throughout childhood, in regards to schoolwork and home life. Once in college a young adult needs to manage his or her time, set and stay within a budget, do laundry, prepare meals, and keep up with academic demands. College life is far less structured than the school days of elementary and high school. Relationships with professors may be less personal due to the larger classroom settings, making it more difficult to get assistance. Prior to enrolling in a college, be sure to do your research to see if the college of interest can meet your needs. Find out about resources available in the school for students with ADHD. Once you start college, consider the following:

- Have realistic expectations.
- Participate in early college activities, such as orientations, get-togethers, etc., in order to meet people in advance.

- Attend all your scheduled classes. It is easy to get behind when classes are skipped.
- Schedule meetings with your professors so they can get to know you.
- Prepare a budget.
- Keep a planner, either on paper or electronically.
- Take a reasonable course load in the first year.
- Get adequate rest and avoid all-nighters.
- Continue your treatment.

If adjusting to college becomes overwhelming, seek assistance right away so that you can add or change your accommodations. Let people know what is happening so they can help you. With support and determination, you can succeed in college.

With support and determination, you can succeed in college.

Liza comments,

At times having ADD was really tough for me. Being educated about my ADD has been very helpful. It helped me understand what was going on in my thought processes. I know what to look for when I am struggling. Medication has made a huge difference in my ability to focus and sustain attention. I know my difficulties and have made accommodations. I am not in a college program that provides Learning Disability Services but I have made the necessary steps to achieve academic success. I study, write papers, and essentially do all my work in the library. I find it to be the only place that I maintain focus. I procrastinate a lot, and thus have devised ways of planning my studies and test preparation skills that prevent me from feeling overwhelmed. Finding a good career match for myself remains to be my most challenging goal.

91. I want to compete in competitive sports in college. Will my medication be detected in routine drug testing?

The National Collegiate Athletic Association (NCAA), as well as national and international athletic federations, bans

121

the use of stimulant medications as possible performance-enhancing substances; however, they also recognize that some students have medically legitimate needs to take stimulant medication. A medical exception procedure has been created that allows for students who are being treated by a physician for ADHD to continue their medication. An application needs to be made to the Drug Education and Drug Testing Subcommittee of the NCAA Committee on Competitive Safeguards and Medical Aspects of Sports. You can apply after testing positive for amphetamine or methylphenidate, but the medical evidence provided needs to document that the diagnosis was made and medication prescribed prior to the positive drug test. It would be more prudent to apply for the exception in advance of drug testing so that unnecessary complications do not arise. Note that a positive drug test for stimulant medication in the absence of a medical exception will result in suspension.

92. Can someone with ADHD join the military?

It may be possible to join the military even with a diagnosis of ADHD. Numerous eligibility criteria for joining the military must be met which fall into the two main categories of skills and aptitude for military service and physical standards. Assessment of aptitude is done via a timed test called the Armed Services Vocational Aptitude Battery. This test examines knowledge in science, mathematics, word knowledge and paragraph comprehension, auto and shop information, mechanics, and electronics. Accommodations are not permitted for this test, so the impact of your ADHD here would depend upon your need for testing accommodations. Physical standards must be met and are evaluated via a complete medical/psychiatric history and physical examination. Conditions that could result in a separation from duty or a medical waiver are identified. The standard in which ADHD becomes an issue are the directives that cite personality, conduct, or behavior disorders that have resulted in impulsiveness and instability as demonstrated by problems with adjustment in school and in work, which would therefore be considered a potential interference with adjustment in the armed services. Additionally cited are the presence of specific academic skills defects and the necessity to use medication to improve academic skills as exclusions. Individual military services may grant waivers to individuals who do not meet the basic eligibility criteria, meaning that you may be able to obtain a waiver if you are able to demonstrate success for a period of time in school or work without the use of medication. Documentation of any treatment of ADHD within the previous three years must be submitted in advance of the medical evaluation. While it may seem unfair that the need for a daily medication is an exclusion, there are many other medical conditions that require daily medication and thus result in exclusion, such as asthma, diabetes, arthritis, and many others. If you are interested in a military career, it is still worthwhile to check with a recruiter as to the possibility of applying and then, if rejected, to ask for a medical waiver. It is best to be up front about your condition so that if accepted it is done under full disclosure.

93. What sorts of jobs are good for people with ADHD?

As with anyone, people with ADHD have differing personalities and interests and thus there are not specific kinds of jobs that are always well suited to someone with ADHD. People with ADHD do tend to switch jobs more often, which can be a function of boredom, risk taking, impulsivity, or interpersonal problems with co-workers, among other things. That said, it is important to choose a job or career in something that you like, as something that holds little interest for you would be very difficult to manage with ADHD. It is easier to capitalize on your strengths in a job that you enjoy. For individuals who tend to be hyperactive and feel the need to keep moving, it is likely best to stay away from jobs that require a lot of sitting or have a lot of down time. You may also find that a job that does not require significant periods of concentration on one thing would be easier to manage. You can also make a job work for you by considering ways to create your own accommodations. Some people find that with their ADHD they do better in a highly structured setting to keep them on task, whereas others prefer loosely structured work environments in which they can express creativity or work at their own pace. Jobs with more immediate and enjoyable consequences are often well suited to ADHD individuals, and self-employment is often preferred.

On the job, you may choose to tell your employer about your ADHD or not, but you should consider making your own accommodations to feel productive and satisfied with your work. Such strategies include:

- Job restructuring
- Keeping a nondistracting workspace
- Working at home
- Obtaining extra clerical support
- Asking that instructions be written as well as verbal
- Obtaining a private office to close out distractions
- Creating uninterrupted blocks of time during the day
- Keeping a notepad during the day to write down information that needs remembering
- Avoiding overscheduling of the day
- Holding something in your hands during meetings to keep them busy

Rather than being viewed solely as disabilities, many aspects of ADHD can be viewed as potential strengths.

The key is to work in a job you enjoy and then build your own accommodations to foster your success. Career or job coaches can be helpful if it is difficult to pin down a job of interest.

94. I am worried I won't succeed due to my ADHD.

Rather than being viewed solely as disabilities, many aspects of ADHD can be viewed as potential strengths. Adults with ADHD can lead productive, fulfilling, and successful lives.

ADHD affects people from all professions and across all walks of life, including well-known people in business and the arts, as well as authors, entertainers, athletes, and politicians. The ability to think about problems in a different way, to be quick in decisions, take risks, and go on instinct are traits that enable many to succeed in new ventures, start new businesses, and bring new ideas to society. There are famous historical figures highly suspected of having suffered from ADHD or learning disabilities based upon written accounts of their behavior as well, such as Albert Einstein and Thomas Edison. Many currently famous entrepreneurs, entertainers, and athletes have written about their struggles with ADHD and/or learning disabilities. ADHD does not have to be a limitation to achieving success.

ADHD affects people from all professions and across all walks of life, including well-known people in business and the arts, as well as authors, entertainers, athletes, and politicians.

95. Should I tell my employer about my ADHD?

Many employers are the ones actually paying the medical bills through contracts established with health insurance companies. As a result they often feel entitled to know what they are paying for. Additionally, if you take time off work related to your condition, you may be concerned about what will be released to your employer to justify the time off. Finally, in many job application forms the issue of a mental disability comes up as part of the application process. All of these issues may lead to concern that your employer will gain knowledge of your illness and negative consequences will result from such knowledge. While all of these issues are of concern, paying the bill does not give an employer the right to specific information beyond the minimum amount necessary. They are on a "need to know" basis. They have no right to know your diagnosis, whether it is medical or psychiatric, for either payment or time away from work. An employer may request information on whether or not the illness will impact on your job performance in any way in order to know if you should remain out of work, or return with a change or reduction in workload. Know that while the American Disabilities Act

Living with ADHD

(ADA) prohibits discrimination in hiring practices for people seeking work, it does not mandate that a disabled person be hired. ADHD is a misunderstood disability that can frighten prospective employers if accommodations are requested up front during the interview process. Finally, any application for employment should ask only if you are suffering from a mental disability that would impair your ability to perform your job. You have to decide if your condition would, in fact, impair your ability to perform your assigned duties. There is no reason you need to disclose to a potential employer that you have been treated or continue to receive treatment for ADHD. Once you have a job, if your performance is adversely affected by your ADHD symptoms, consider modifications that can help you improve on your own, such as day planners, timers on your watch, or notepads. Use of a coach can help you establish appropriate accommodations without involving your employer. If you need certain accommodations, you may be able to request them based upon a discussion with your supervisor about things you need to work optimally. If your supervisor is not supportive of your requests, however, you may need to disclose your diagnosis. In doing so you can educate your supervisor about the condition and the type of work environment you need. If still met with resistance, keep in mind that ADHD is considered a protected disability under the ADA. Under this act, an employer is required to make reasonable accommodations for employees with a disability as long as these accommodations do not impose undue hardship on the operation of the business. If you have concerns about discrimination due to your ADHD, consider consultation with an employment attorney.

96. Will medication impair my ability to drive?

To the contrary, there is mounting evidence that medication treatment improves your ability to drive a vehicle. Drivers with untreated ADHD have been found to exhibit significant driving performance deficits. Young drivers are 2 to 4 times more likely to have traffic accidents, 3 times more likely to have injuries, 4 times more likely to be at fault, and 6 to 8 times more likely to have their licenses suspended. In studies, adults with ADHD are noted to have more speeding citations, license suspensions, crashes, and crashes involving bodily injury than controls. In a study using a computer-simulated driving test, ADHD adults were found to have more erratic steering, difficulty steering, and scrapes than controls and also score lower on tests of driving rules and decision making.

Research has also shown that many indices that measure driving performance are improved with the use of medication. Impaired attention and impulsivity are likely both contributory to the impaired driving performance seen in ADHD patients. Evidence of driving impairment highlights the importance of treating ADHD for many reasons other than for academic or work-related purposes and the importance of daily treatment.

Liza comments,

Due to difficulties I have with driving when I am off my medication, I fear that one day my license will be taken away. Being on my medication helps me be a better driver. When I don't take my medication I am more likely to have traffic violations. I have been stopped for speeding several times. I have been to court and have paid a lot of money to lawyers. I now have a radar detector in my car and lower the volume of the music that is played to minimize distraction, and try to be mindful of taking my medication regularly.

97. Will I be able to go off medication?

ADHD is usually a lifelong illness that, if present in adulthood, is not apt to go away (some children and adolescents do not continue to have ADHD into adulthood). Your decision to go off medication will be based upon determining your functioning as well as assessing the best time to have a medication-free trial. Since remission of the disorder does not occur, symptoms will persist when medication is stopped. You may, however, be better equipped during certain life periods to handle symptoms of your ADHD without medication. This is more likely possible if you have been getting therapy to address coping with your symptoms as well as to learn techniques for managing symptoms. Use of a coach to learn specific strategies may facilitate your going off medication. Timing may also affect when and if you choose to stop your medication. Demands may be higher in certain job or relationship situations and, with those demands, it can be more difficult to utilize behavioral strategies for your symptoms. You may decide to go off medication for a certain time period, and then resume it if functioning declines again due to your symptoms.

Samantha comments,

I don't have concerns about whether or not I can go off the medication. I am happy to have medication that can effectively assist me in managing my symptoms and cannot imagine choosing to stop my treatment. On days that I miss my medication, I recognize the increased difficulty I have in functioning both at work and at home, and this is an unpleasant feeling.

Liza comments,

Right now I am doing well on my medication. If my symptoms impair my functioning then I will stay on them. If I can manage without medications in the future, I will go off of them.

As a group, people with ADHD have many positive traits that can be attributed to their active, impulsive minds.

98. Are there advantageous aspects to ADHD?

The diagnosis of ADHD should not be viewed as entirely negative. As a group, people with ADHD have many positive traits that can be attributed to their active, impulsive minds. While the traits listed here are not necessarily applicable to all individuals with ADHD, they are traits that many people have noted to occur in those people with whom they treat, work, live, and associate. These traits are:

- Creativity
- Spontaneity
- High energy level
- Sense of humor
- Resiliency
- Compassion
- Novelty-seeking
- Intuitiveness
- Willingness to take risks
- Enthusiasm
- Flexibility
- Forgiving
- Quick-thinking

If these traits are familiar (either in yourself or in someone you care about), keep them in mind when the frustrating aspects of ADHD start to bring you down!

Samantha comments,

The up side of ADHD includes having the ability to multitask, having a great sense of humor, leading an un-boring life, having an aggressive stance that some call "pushy," and having a great desire for adventure and passion in life. I am not fearful to explore or challenge myself as I have the impulsivity to jump into things without thinking too much. I am not shy and am very vocal. I have few friends but many acquaintances. I love my life.

Liza comments,

I have always had friends. I am creative and very spontaneous. I have always loved entertaining people and have sense of humor. I am always ready to talk and I can talk a lot. I have been told that I have a great personality and am very mature for my age. I also require less sleep and can get more done.

99. What is CHADD? How can they help?

Children and Adults with Attention-Deficit/Hyperactivity Disorder (CHADD), is a national non-profit organization that provides education, advocacy, and support for individuals with ADHD. In addition to keeping a website, CHADD publishes a variety of printed materials to keep members and professionals current on research advances, medications, and treatments affecting individuals with ADHD. These materials include the ATTENTION! magazine; the CHADD Information and Resource Guide to ADHD; News From CHADD; a free, electronically mailed current events newsletter; as well as other publications of specific interest to educators, professionals, and parents.

CHADD was founded in 1987, at which time there were very few places to obtain support or information. From one parent support group in Florida, the organization grew dramatically to become the leading nonprofit national organization for children and adults with ADHD.

The goals of CHADD are to serve as a clearinghouse for evidence-based information on ADHD, to serve as a local face-to-face family support group for families and individuals affected by ADHD, and to serve as an advocate for appropriate public policies and public recognition in response to needs faced by families and individuals with ADHD. CHADD publishes a magazine called ATTENTION! and currently has 235 chapters in 43 states and Puerto Rico. Chapter meetings are coordinated by volunteers and typically held in persons' homes. There is a website, www.chadd.org, that can provide further information and resources for those interested in becoming involved in their local chapters.

100. Where can I find out more information about ADHD?

It is not possible to discuss all possible aspects of ADHD in one small volume. The Appendix that follows contains information about organizations, websites, and publications that can be useful to patients with ADHD and their families.

Living with ADHD

Appendix

Organizations

Attention Deficit Disorder Association
PO Box 7557
Wilmington, DE 19803-9997
(800) 939-1019
www.add.org

Children and Adults with Attention-Deficit/Hyperactivity Disorder
8181 Professional Place, Suite 150
Landover, MD 20785
(301) 306-7070
www.chadd.org

Disability Rights Education & Defense Fund
2212 Sixth Street
Berkeley, CA 94710
(800) 348-4232
www.dredf.org

Food and Drug Administration
10903 New Hampshire Avenue
Silver Spring, MD 20903
(888) INFO-FDA
www.fda.gov

Mental Health America
2000 North Beauregard Street, 6th Floor
Alexandria, VA 22311
(800) 969-NMHA
www.nmha.org

National Alliance on Mental Illness
2107 Wilson Boulevard, Suite 300
Arlington, VA 22201-3042
(703) 524-7600
www.nami.org

National Institute of Mental Health
Science Writing, Press, and Dissemination Branch
6001 Executive Boulevard, Room 8184, MSC 9663
Bethesda, MD 20892-9663
(866) 615-6464
www.nimh.nih.gov

Websites

www.aacap.org
American Academy of Child and Adolescent Psychiatry website with resources
for patients and their families

www.abct.org
Association for Behavioral and Cognitive Therapies website with link to find
a therapist

www.aboutourkids.org
NYU Child Study Center website on child mental health

www.academyofct.org
Academy of Cognitive Therapy website with links for consumer information and
finding a certified cognitive therapist

www.aetonline.org
Association of Educational Therapists website at which you can learn more about
educational therapy as well as information on finding an educational therapist

www.apahelpcenter.org
American Psychological Association website with articles and information
for consumers

www.bazelon.org
Bazelon Center for Mental Health Law website with information pertaining to their work in national legal advocacy for the mentally ill

www.dr-bob.org
Psychopharmacology tips

www.eeoc.gov
U.S. Equal Employment Opportunity Commission website with information regarding the American Disabilities Act

www.healthfinder.gov
U.S. Department of Health and Human Services-sponsored website that connects to resources on the web pertaining to health-related information.

www.healthyminds.org
American Psychiatric Association website with public information on various mental health topics

www.mentalhealth.org
U.S. Department of Health and Human Services website for mental health information

www.nacbt.org
National Association of Cognitive-Behavioral Therapists website with information for consumers and link to find a certified cognitive-behavioral therapist

www.naswdc.org/resources
National Association of Social Workers website with listing of social workers meeting national standards

www.webmd.com
Website providing medical and health and wellness information

Glossary

A

Addiction: Continued use of a mood-altering substance despite physical, psychological, or social harm. It is characterized by a lack of control in the amount and frequency of use, cravings, continued use in the presence of adverse effects, denial of negative consequences, and a tendency to abuse other mood-altering substances.

Adoption study: A scientific study designed to control for genetic relatedness and environmental influences by comparing siblings adopted into different families.

Agonist: A drug that binds to the receptor of a cell and triggers a response by the cell.

Alternative treatment: A treatment for a medical condition that has not undergone scientific studies to demonstrate its efficacy.

Anterior cingulate gyrus: A part of the limbic system of the brain that is involved in emotional formation and processing, learning, and memory.

Antidepressant: A drug specifically marketed for and capable of relieving the symptoms of clinical depression. It is often used to treat conditions other than depression.

Antipsychotic: A drug that treats psychotic symptoms, such as hallucinations, delusions, and thought disorders. Antipsychotics can be used to treat certain mood disorders as well.

Arousal: A state of responsiveness to sensory stimulation or excitability.

Augmentation: In pharmacotherapy, a strategy of using a second medication to enhance the positive effects of an existing medication in the regimen.

Automatic thoughts: Thoughts that occur spontaneously whenever a specific, common event occurs in one's life, and that are often associated with depression.

Axon: A single fiber of a nerve cell through which a message is sent via an electrical impulse to a receiving neuron. Each nerve cell has one axon.

B

Basal ganglia: A region of the brain consisting of three groups of nerve cells (called the caudate nucleus, putamen, and the globus pallidus) that are collectively responsible for control of movement. Abnormalities in the basal ganglia can result in involuntary movement disorders.

Bipolar depression: An episode of depression that occurs in the course of bipolar disorder.

Bipolar disorder: A mental illness defined by episodes of mania or hypomania, classically alternating with episodes of depression. However, the condition can take various forms, such as repeated episodes of mania only or a lack of alternating episodes.

C

Catastrophic thinking: A type of automatic thought during which the individual quickly assumes the worst outcome for a given situation.

Catecholamines: Amines that are derived from tyrosine and function as hormones, neurotransmitters, or both.

Central nervous system: Nerve cells and their support cells in the brain and spinal cord.

Cerebral cortex: The outer portion of the brain, which is comprised of gray matter and made up of numerous folds that greatly increase the surface area of the brain. Advanced motor function, social abilities, language, and problem solving are coordinated in this area of the brain.

Coaching: A practice of helping clients determine and achieve personal goals.

Cognitions: The mental processes of knowing, thinking, learning, and judging.

Cognitive behavioral therapy: A combination of cognitive and behavioral approaches in psychotherapy, during which the therapist focuses on automatic thoughts and behavior of a self-defeating quality in order to make one more conscious of them

and replace them with more positive thoughts and behaviors.

Comorbid: The presence of two or more mental disorders, such as depression and anxiety.

Compliance: Extent that behavior follows medical advice, such as by taking prescribed treatments. Compliance can refer to medications as well as to appointments and psychotherapy sessions.

Concordance: In genetics, a similarity in a twin pair with respect to presence or absence of illness.

Contingency contracting: A behavioral therapy technique that utilizes reinforcers or rewards to modify behavior.

Countertransference: The attitudes, opinions, and behaviors that a therapist attributes to his or her patient, not based on the true nature of the patient but rather the biased nature of the therapist because the patient reminds the therapist of his or her own past relationships.

D

Dependence: The body's reliance on a drug to function normally. Physical dependence results in withdrawal when the drug is stopped suddenly. Dependence should be contrasted to addiction.

Depression: A medical condition associated with changes in thoughts, moods, and behaviors.

Developmental disorder: One of several disorders that interrupt normal development in childhood; a developmental disorder may affect a single area of development or several.

Discontinuation syndrome: Physical symptoms that occur when a drug is suddenly stopped.

Dopamine: A catecholamine that serves as a neurotransmitter in the brain.

Dyslexia: A reading disability that alters the way the brain processes written material; such a disability is neurological in origin.

Dysthymic disorder: A type of depressive disorder that is characterized by the presence of chronic, mild depressive symptoms.

E

Educational therapy: An education intervention that investigates, defines, and addresses an individual's pattern of learning.

EEG biofeedback: A learning strategy that enables persons to alter their brain waves.

Effect size: In research, indices that measure the magnitude of a treatment response.

Efficacy: The capacity to produce a desired effect, such as the performance of a drug or therapy in relieving symptoms of depression such as feeling down, trouble concentrating, etc.

Electrocardiogram: A noninvasive recording of the electrical activity of the heart.

Electrochemically: The mechanism by which signals are transmitted neurologically. Brain chemicals, or neurotransmitters, alter the electrical conductivity of nerve tissue, causing a signal to be transmitted or sent.

Endorphins: Chemicals produced by the body that serve to suppress pain.

Enzyme: A protein made in the body that serves to break down or create other molecules. Enzymes serve as catalysts to biochemical reactions in the body.

Euthymic: To be characterized by moderation of mood.

Executive functions: A set of cognitive abilities that control and regulate other abilities and behaviors.

F

Fight or flight: A reaction in the body that occurs in response to an immediate threat. Adrenaline is released, which allows for rapid energy to face the threat (fight) or to run (flight).

First-degree relative: Immediate biologically related family member, such as biological parents or full siblings.

Flooding: A behavioral therapy technique that involves exposure to the maximal level of anxiety as quickly as possible.

Free association: The mental process of saying aloud whatever comes to mind, suppressing the natural tendency to censor or filter thoughts. This is a technique used in psychoanalysis and in psychodynamic psychotherapy.

Functional: Pertaining to the ability to perform day-to-day responsibilities, such as in one's work, home, and school lives.

G

Genetic: Of or relating to genes, the DNA sequence that codes for a specific protein or that regulates other genes. That which is genetic is heritable.

Graded exposure: A psychotherapeutic technique applied to rid a patient of specific phobias. A gradual exposure to the phobic situation is set about first through imagery techniques and then with limited exposure in time and intensity before full exposure occurs.

Grandiosity: The tendency to consider the self or one's ideas better than or superior to what is reality.

Gray matter: The part of the brain that contains the nerve cell bodies, including the cell nucleus and its metabolic machinery, as opposed to the axons, which are essentially the "transmission wires" of the nerve cell. The cerebral cortex contains gray matter.

H

Half-life: The time it takes for half of the blood concentration of a medication to be eliminated from the body. Half-life also determines the time to equilibrium of a drug in the blood and the frequency of dosing to achieve that equilibrium.

Heritability: The proportion of observed variation of a particular trait that is attributable to genetic factors in contrast to environmental factors.

Hormonal: Referring to the chemicals that are secreted by the endocrine glands (the thyroid, pancreas, pituitary glands, and others) and act throughout the body.

Hyperfocus: Intense mental concentration on or visualization of a narrow subject.

Hyperkinesis: Hyperactivity; excessive motor movement.

Hyperpyrexia: Abnormally high fever.

Hypertensive crisis: A condition characterized by extremely high blood pressure levels.

Hypomania: A milder form of mania with the same symptoms but of lesser intensity.

Hypothyroidism: Decrease in or absence of thyroid hormone, which is secreted by an endocrine gland near the throat and has wide metabolic effects.

I

Insomnia: A condition marked by the inability to fall asleep, middle of the night awakening, or early morning awakening.

Interpersonal therapy: A form of therapy. Unlike psychodynamic therapy that focuses on developmental relationships, interpersonal therapy focuses strictly on current relationships and conflicts within them.

J

Jaundice: Yellow staining of the skin and sclerae of the eyes due to abnormally high levels of bilirubin, which typically indicates liver or gallbladder disease.

L

Locus ceruleus: An area within the brainstem with neurons that synthesize norepinephrine and from where axon projections spread widely throughout the central nervous system.

M

Mania: A condition characterized by elevation of mood (extreme euphoria or irritability) associated with racing thoughts, decreased need for sleep, hyperactivity, and poor impulse control. One episode of mania (in the absence of an ingested substance) is needed to diagnose bipolar disorder.

Mental illness: A medical condition defined by functional symptoms with as yet no specific pathophysiology that impairs social, academic, and occupational function.

Mental status: A snapshot portrait of one's cognitive and emotional functioning at a particular point in time. It is always included as part of a psychiatric examination.

Metabolize: The process of breaking down a drug in the blood.

Midbrain: The part of the brainstem that is responsible for basic, unconscious body functions.

Modeling: Learning that occurs from observation.

Mood disorder: A type of mental illness that affects mood primarily and cognition secondarily. Mood disorders predominantly consist of depression and bipolar disorder.

Mood stabilizer: Typically refers to medications used for the treatment and prevention of mood swings, such as those from depression and mania.

Motor cortex: Portion of the cerebral cortex that is directly related to voluntary movement. Also known as the motor strip, its anatomy correlates accurately with specific bodily movements, such as moving the left upper or lower extremities.

N

Neurobiological: Of or relating to the biological study of the nervous system.

Neuroimaging: The use of techniques to create an image of the structure or function of the brain; CT scans and brain MRIs are examples.

Neurological: Referring to all matters of the nervous system that include the brain, brainstem, spinal cord, and peripheral nerves. Problems with specific, identifiable, pathophysiologic processes are generally considered to be neurological as opposed to psychiatric. Problems with elements of both pathophysiological and psychiatric manifestations are considered to be neuropsychiatric.

Neuron: A nerve cell made up of a cell body with extensions called the dendrites and the axon. The dendrites carry messages from the synapse to the cell body, and the axon carries messages to the synapse to communicate with other nerve cells.

Neurophysiology: The part of science devoted specifically to the physiology of the nervous system.

Neuropsychological testing: The assessment of brain functioning through structured and systematic behavioral observation.

Neurotransmitter: Chemical in the brain that is released by nerve cells to send a message to other cells via the cell receptors.

Norepinephrine: A neurotransmitter that is involved in the regulation of mood, arousal, and memory.

O

Off-label: Prescribing of a medication for indications other than those outlined by the Food and Drug Administration.

Overgeneralization: The act of taking a specific event, usually one that was psychologically traumatic, and applying one's reactions to that event to an ever-increasing array of events that are not really in the same class but are perceived as such.

P

Parietal lobe: A lobe in the brain that integrates sensory information from different modalities from various parts of the body.

Peripheral nervous system: The part of the nervous system that constitutes nerves outside of the brain and the spinal cord, such as nerves that innervate the limbs.

Personality disorder: Maladaptive behavior patterns that persist throughout the life span, causing functional impairments.

Petit mal: A type of seizure characterized by brief, unpredictable lapses in consciousness; also known as absence seizures.

Pharmacokinetic: The process by which a drug is absorbed, distributed, metabolized, and eliminated by the body.

Pharmacological: Pertaining to all chemicals that, when ingested, cause a physiological process to occur in the body. Psychopharmacologic refers to those physiologic processes that have direct psychological effects.

Physiological: Pertaining to functions and activities of the living matter, such as organs, tissues, or cells.

Placebo: An inert substance that, when ingested, causes absolutely no physiological process to occur but may have psychological effects.

Positive reinforcement: The presentation of something rewarding or pleasurable immediately following a behavior that makes it more likely the behavior will occur again.

Prefrontal lobe: The anterior part of the cerebral cortex that is implicated in planning complex cognitive actions.

Pressured speech: Characterized by the need to keep speaking; it is difficult to interrupt someone with this type of speech. This is commonly seen in manic or hypomanic mood states.

Presynaptic: That part of a nerve cell that is proximal to the synapse.

Prevalence: Ratio of the frequency of cases in the population in a given time period of a particular event to the number of persons in the population at risk for the event.

Projection: The attribution of one's own unconscious thoughts and feelings to others.

Psychodynamic: Referring to a type of therapy that focuses on one's interpersonal relationships, developmental experiences, and the transference relationship with his or her therapist.

Psychological testing: The use of samples of behavior to infer generalizations about a given individual.

Psychomotor agitation: Hyperactive or restless movement. It can be seen in highly anxious states, manic mood states, or intoxicated states.

Psychopharmacologist: A specialist in the study of actions, effects, and development of psychoactive medications.

Psychosocial: Pertaining to environmental circumstances that can impact one's psychological well-being.

Psychotic: Relating to the loss of contact with reality, which can be characterized by the presence of hallucinations or delusions.

Q

QT interval: A measurement on electrocardiogram that represents the total duration of electrical activity of the ventricles of the heart; abnormal QT intervals may be evidence for increased risk of abnormal heart rhythms.

R

Receptor: A protein on a cell to which specific chemicals from within the body or from the environment bind in order to cause changes in the cell that result in an electrochemical message for a certain action to be taken by that cell.

Remission: Complete cessation of all symptoms associated with a specific mental illness, which can be temporary or permanent.

Resistance: The tendency to avoid treatment interventions, often unconsciously (e.g., missed appointments, arriving late, forgetting medication).

Response inhibition: In behavioral therapy, the weakening of a response to a given stimulus.

Reuptake: The reabsorption of a substance by the cell that originally released the substance.

S

Schema: The internal representation of the world that each person holds, which can be revised as new information is obtained.

Serotonin: A neurotransmitter found in the brain and throughout the body. Serotonin is involved in mood regulation, anxiety, pain perception, appetite, sleep, sexual behavior, and impulsive behavior.

Serotonin syndrome: An extremely rare but life-threatening syndrome associated with the direct physiological effects of serotonin overload on the body. Symptoms include flushing, high fever, tachycardia, and seizures.

Stressors: Environmental influences on the body and mind that can have gradual adverse effects.

Sympathomimetic: Mimics the effects of stimulation of organs and structures by the sympathetic nervous system.

Synaptic cleft: The junction between two neurons where neurotransmitters are released, resulting in the transmission of a message between the two neurons.

T

Thalamus: A region in the brain that has multiple functions including the relay of information to the cerebral cortex and regulating arousal, awareness, and activity.

Transference: The unconscious assignment of feelings and attitudes to a therapist from previous important relationships in one's life (parents and siblings). The relationship follows the pattern of its prototype and can be either negative or positive. The transference relationship is a critical event for the progress of a patient in psychodynamic therapy.

Transporter: A protein that travels through a cell membrane into a cell, carrying specific nutrients, ions, or chemicals with it.

Treatment plan: The plan agreed on by patient and clinician that will be implemented to treat a mental illness. It incorporates all modalities (therapy and medication).

U

Unconscious: An underlying motivation for behavior that has developed over the course of life experience and is not available to the conscious or thoughtful mind.

Utilization behavior: A condition in which a person has difficulty resisting the impulse to pick up or manipulate objects within his or her visual field or reach.

W

White matter: Tracts in the brain that consist of sheaths (called myelin) covering long nerve fibers.

Working memory: A system in the brain for temporarily storing and managing information required to carry out complex cognitive tasks.

Index